The 5:2 Diet Cookbook

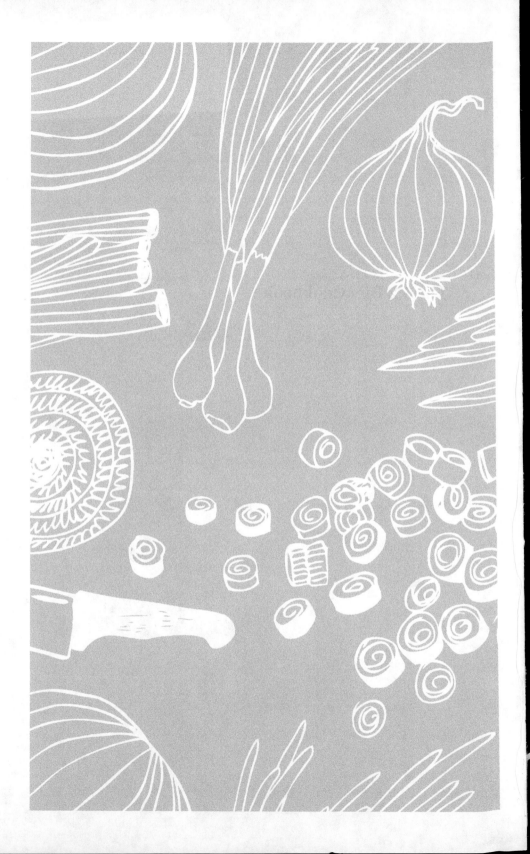

The 5:2 Diet Cookbook

OVER 75 FAST DIET RECIPES AND
MEAL PLANS TO LOSE WEIGHT WITH
INTERMITTENT FASTING

MENDOCINO PRESS

Contents

Introduction

Have you ever tried to lose weight by starving yourself for weeks on end, and finally quit in defeat because you felt deprived, exhausted, and downright grumpy? You're not alone. Although cutting calories is a viable strategy for weight loss, most people quit eating plans based on calorie restriction because they simply cannot do it day after day (after day!), even when the diet is successful.

The 5:2 Diet is based on the concept of *intermittent fasting*. The diet features two calorie-restricted days and then allows you to eat normal quantities of food for the other five days of the week. Imagine just two days of eating about one-quarter of your usual amount of food, sandwiched between non-fasting days. You can still enjoy all your favorite foods most of the time and lose weight. The 5:2 Diet can also reduce your risk of chronic diseases such as heart disease and diabetes.

The 5:2 Diet is a sustainable lifestyle choice because it doesn't really require drastic changes to your routine, expensive foods, or meal replacements. That's the beauty of it. You might even be fasting already without realizing it! If you eat dinner around six without snacking afterward, and then dash out the door in the morning to start your day, that's about sixteen hours of fasting before you have your first snack midmorning. Most people fast to some extent, and the 5:2 Diet simply makes it part of your routine rather than a by-product of a busy schedule. This book is a great blueprint for the 5:2 Diet, and you'll even have seventy-seven delicious recipes that can be used on non-fasting days as well.

To help you get a full understanding of the 5:2 Diet, this book is organized to walk you through the information step by step. By the time you reach the delicious recipes in Part Two, you'll be perfectly prepared to start fasting! Some of the important takeaways from this book will include:

- Comprehensive knowledge of the 5:2 Diet, as well as the history of the plan and fasting
- Essential information about the health benefits of the 5:2 Diet and the science behind it

- What to expect in the first month, simple strategies for transitioning to the 5:2 plan, and ten steps to get you started
- Answers to common questions that come up when people start the 5:2 Diet
- Handy information about foods to eat on fasting days, as well as those to avoid, along with low-calorie cooking tips for preparing all your meals
- Meal plans that use many recipes in this book for your first month, and show exactly what five hundred and six hundred calories look like on your fasting days
- Advice on what approach you might want to take on your non-fasting days

With this book in hand, you'll have a detailed roadmap for your journey on the 5:2 Diet. Here's to your success!

PART ONE

The 5:2 Diet

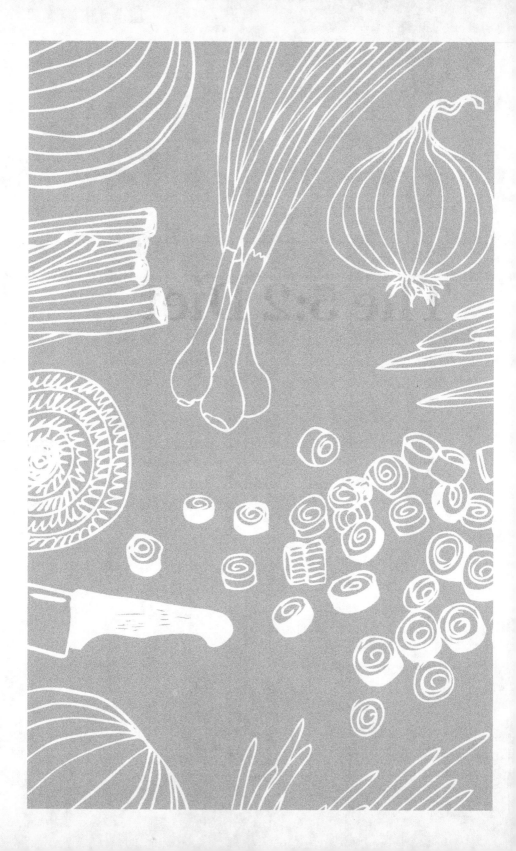

CHAPTER ONE

Basics of the 5:2 Diet

There seems to be a new fad diet every week that touts the benefits of some obscure herb found in far-flung jungles or promises weight loss if you give up every food group but one for the rest of your life. Since obesity and chronic diseases are so prevalent, any solution that strikes a chord or offers hope seems worth trying. Yet these fads often fail because they have no foundation based on fact.

The principles behind the 5:2 Diet are set solidly on data drawn from centuries of fasting by almost every civilization in the world and irrefutable scientific research. The 5:2 Diet is the last diet you'll ever have to try in the quest for better health because it's a realistic lifestyle choice that is sustainable and produces results. It will simply become part of your everyday life.

WHAT IS THE 5:2 DIET?

The 5:2 Diet, also known as the Fast Diet and intermittent fasting, is an extremely popular eating plan that combines two calorie-restricted days (fasts) with five regular eating days in a week. The fasting days do not involve complete food deprivation, but rather eating about a quarter of what is considered to be normal calorie consumption in a day. This eating plan is supposed to help followers lose weight and experience many of the health benefits linked to fasting.

So how did fasting become a mainstream diet plan? In 2012, a medical journalist in the United Kingdom named Michael Mosley lost twenty pounds after trying the 5:2 combination of intermittent fasting. His success and the resulting media storm inspired TV shows and books, which in turn motivated many people to try this lifestyle change. The positive buzz on the 5:2 Diet continued to grow as people lost weight, felt better, and found the diet easier to commit to than standard weeklong calorie-restriction diets. The 5:2 Diet is flexible enough to make it practical, does not require radical food or cooking changes, and it works.

The basic guidelines of the 5:2 Diet are very straightforward:

- Combine five regular eating days and two days of fasting each week.
- Fasting days should not be consecutive.
- On fasting days, consume a maximum of five hundred calories if you are a woman and six hundred calories if you are a man.
- There are no food restrictions or schedules on fasting days except the calorie allotment. You can eat six small meals, three moderate meals, or one large meal, depending on your preference.
- On non-fasting days, eat anything you want, but try to keep your calories to 2,000 per day (women) or 2,600 per day (men), and stick to whole foods like vegetables, fruits, and whole grains whenever feasible.
- Make sure you drink at least eight glasses of water per day.

THE HISTORY BEHIND THE 5:2 DIET

Fasting is certainly not a new concept, and it wouldn't be far-fetched to assume early mankind fasted out of necessity due to a scarcity of food. Fasting on purpose has been practiced for centuries by many cultures for religious and healing purposes. Great thinkers such as Hippocrates, Aristotle, and Plato recommended fasting for mental clarity and to promote revitalization of the body. Hippocrates, considered to be the father of modern medicine, is thought to have advocated short fasts for patients with arthritis, digestive complaints, and colds. Fasting is meant to let the body rest and detoxify without having to expend the energy that is required to digest and process food.

Most current religions in the world have used fasting for sacrifice, spiritual clarity, purification, and penance for sins or failings. Fasting is meant to show a commitment to the spiritual while ignoring the physical needs of the body. Religions that use fasting in some form are:

- Buddhism
- Christianity (including Catholicism and Lutheranism)
- Hinduism
- Islam
- Judaism
- North American Indian

Fasting has also been used as a political statement by people like Mahatma Gandhi, who fasted to promote passive resistance and encourage peace among peoples. Other groups since Gandhi have embraced this method for their own causes with mixed results.

Healers, mystics, and religions still recommend fasting for health purposes, but traditional (Western) medicine has taken a little time to catch up and embrace the practice. Sometimes religion and science cooperate to produce studies like one documenting improved blood pressure and cholesterol levels with fasting during Ramadan (Nematy 2012). Research has been done on the effects of fasting with respect to weight loss, heart disease, diabetes, and other diseases with interesting results (Brown 2013). It is this kind of research that spurred British medical journalist Michael Mosley to experiment with fasting in order to lose some weight and improve his cholesterol, blood sugar, and blood pressure levels.

Mosley tried several different variations of fasting, including a complete fast, before settling on a two-day fast combined with five days of normal eating. This combination eventually produced a twenty-pound weight loss and improved numbers on all of his medical tests. Thus, the 5:2 Diet was born! It took a British television show called *Eat, Fast, and Live Longer*, which aired in 2012, to really bring this diet plan to the mainstream. Fasting is now an accepted diet in the United Kingdom and is starting to become popular throughout many countries.

THE SCIENCE BEHIND THE 5:2 DIET

Fasting and its effects on the body have been the focus of many studies and much research, mostly on animals, and the results seem to link fasting to numerous health benefits. This is the reason why Mosley created the 5:2 Diet and why people all over the world have embraced it. Weight loss, lower cholesterol and blood pressure, and a reduced risk of diabetes and cardiovascular disease are just some of the reasons you might want to try the 5:2 Diet. The science supporting the practice of fasting is quite compelling, and the accumulation of facts is very convincing.

People haven't always had such an abundance of food available twenty-four hours a day like they do now. Studies that look at genes and processes in the body show that the human body has adapted to deal with situations of food scarcity, and this adaptation can be used to promote weight loss and health improvements through fasting. Here are some of the changes that occur in the body when you fast:

- When you intermittently fast, a gene known as "the skinny gene" or SIRT1 is triggered in the body. This gene inhibits fat storage and encourages cell repair and maintenance (Allard 2009).
- Fasting lowers the production of a protein called insulin-like growth factor 1 (IGF-1), which is linked to the development of chronic diseases such as cancer and heart disease, as well as aging in higher levels (Fontana 2008).
- Studies have shown that fasting lowers cholesterol levels and blood pressure (Nematy 2012).
- Other studies have documented improved blood sugar levels, increased longevity, and a reduced risk of heart disease, diabetes, and neurological diseases (Brown 2013).
- When the body does not have to process food constantly, the pancreas can rest, which leads to increased insulin sensitivity and a reduced risk of obesity and diabetes (Hughes 1984).
- Fasting changes the environment in the body, which can limit the adaptation potential of cancer cells. The growth of five to eight types of cancer was slowed after a forty-eight-hour fast in animal studies conducted at the University of Southern California in 2009 (Raffaghello 2010).
- Fasting for forty-eight hours after chemotherapy doubled survival rates in lab animals, and preliminary human studies showed that patients experienced fewer side effects if they fasted after chemotherapy (Raffaghello 2010).
- Fasting can decrease the oxidative damage done by free radicals because it increases the stress resistance in cells, which can reduce the risk of cancer (Sohal 1996).
- Studies conducted over many years on people who eat 30 percent fewer calories than normal show less cancer, obesity, inflammation, heart disease, and diabetes (Fontana 2004).
- Fasting for as little as sixteen hours increases the level of a protein called brain-derived neurotropic factor (BDNF) by between 50 and 400 percent. BDNF is essential for memory and learning, and it protects the brain from changes in the cells linked to dementia, Parkinson's, and Alzheimer's disease (Mattson 2005).
- The progression of the metabolic and neuropathological abnormalities linked with Huntington's disease is slowed with fasting in animal studies (Wenzhen 2003).

HEALTH BENEFITS OF THE 5:2 DIET

Most of the people trying the 5:2 Diet aren't usually looking for mental clarity or spiritual awareness, because those goals involve a different type of fasting technique. The main reason people embark on the 5:2 Diet is to lose weight or to get healthier. There are many health improvements associated with intermittent fasting that you can experience after following the diet for a few weeks. Once the body begins to react positively to a fasting schedule, the 5:2 Diet will benefit you in the following ways:

- Promotes weight loss
- Detoxifies the body
- Improves inflammatory conditions
- Reduces the risk of some cancers
- Helps prevent cardiovascular disease
- Reduces cholesterol levels
- Improves response to chemotherapy
- Enhances cognitive function
- Reduces blood sugar
- Decreases blood pressure
- Eliminates food cravings
- Reduces the risk of—and in some cases reverses—type 2 diabetes
- Improves immunity
- Helps with addictions
- Lowers systemwide inflammation
- Improves insulin resistance
- Boosts metabolism
- Slows the aging process and reduces the risk of age-related diseases such as dementia
- Increases life span
- Slows the progress of Huntington's disease
- Improves pancreatic function

Now that you've learned the background and some basics of the 5:2 Diet, read on for answers to common questions, lists of foods to enjoy and to avoid, and other essential information to guide you toward your diet goals.

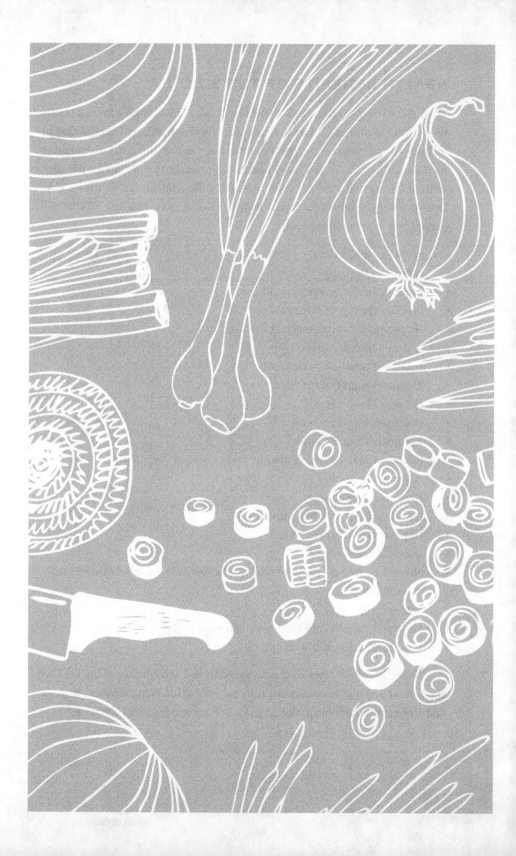

CHAPTER TWO

Getting Started with the 5:2 Diet

When you want to make a life change like addressing a health issue or losing weight, it's often difficult to create a plan instead of jumping right in. Although enthusiasm and commitment are wonderful, unforeseen practical hurdles or unanswered questions can easily derail the best intentions to change. So even if you're convinced that the 5:2 Diet is the right choice for you, take the time to read about how to get started on the plan, what you'll be eating, and what you can expect in the first month of fasting. You might have to change some parts of your routine, cooking techniques, and the types of food in your fridge and pantry. These changes shouldn't be too great because you'll be eating "normally" for most of the week, but it's better to have a complete understanding of the 5:2 Diet before starting.

5:2 DIET FAQS

Whether you're a fasting beginner or have been on the 5:2 Diet for a few weeks, you'll probably have some questions about the plan. Here are some of the common ones.

Will I be hungry?

Yes. You will experience moments of hunger during the 5:2 Diet, but they won't be physically debilitating. Keep in mind that hunger is often thirst in disguise, so take a drink of water to see if the feeling abates before grabbing food. You can plan your fasting meals to ensure your hunger isn't too extreme by adding lots of filling vegetables to your day.

Does the 5:2 Diet have different effects on men and women?

There are some differences between genders when it comes to fasting. Women usually see no improvement in triglyceride levels, and their HDL (good) cholesterol stays stable. Men will see their triglyceride levels decrease. Studies have also shown that women experience no improvement in insulin sensitivity, while men will see increased sensitivity. Glucose tolerance actually got worse for many women in the study. These results will vary from person to person, though.

Do I have to fast two days in a row?

The recommendation is not to do your fasting days consecutively, nor exceed forty-eight hours in total.

What kinds of side effects can I expect when fasting?

As long as you follow the recommendations of the 5:2 Diet, you shouldn't experience too many side effects, and they will eventually go away after a few weeks on the diet as your body gets used to the new routine. Many of these can be attributed to either dehydration or low blood sugar. Side effects that you might have while on the 5:2 Diet include:

- Bad breath
- Constipation or other digestive distress
- Dizziness
- Fatigue
- Headache
- Hunger
- Insomnia
- Moodiness

Is there a meal schedule on fasting days?

You can eat anything you want on fasting days as long as you stay within the calorie range for your gender. You might want to take your routine into account when deciding on your eating schedule in order to have an easier time getting through the day. For example, if you're grumpy when you skip breakfast, make sure that's one of your meals. If you know your energy slumps in the afternoon, try to allot an energy-packed snack.

Is coffee forbidden when fasting?

You can certainly still have your morning coffee or tea on the 5:2 Diet, but if you're someone who likes cream and sugar in your beverage, those calories will count toward your day's total.

Should I use meal replacements when fasting?

You can choose any food you want on your fasting days. Meal replacement bars and shakes are designed to have very precise calorie counts, so it would be easy to incorporate them. Make sure you choose products meant for weight loss rather than those intended to aid in weight gain for body builders or you could wind up eating a bar with more than three hundred calories!

Can everyone follow the 5:2 Diet?

It's always a good idea to consult your health-care provider before embarking on any diet change, particularly if you have an existing health condition. Some people should not intermittently fast, including those who:

- Are taking warfarin, insulin, or any other medication for a medical condition
- Are underweight or clinically obese
- Are children or teenagers
- Are pregnant or nursing
- Are hypoglycemic
- Have peptic ulcers
- Have a history of eating disorders or an active eating disorder
- Have type 1 diabetes
- Recently had surgery
- Have a compromised immune system

Won't my body go into starvation mode if I fast, and then I'll gain weight?

This is true to an extent, but not within the parameters of the 5:2 Diet. Studies have shown that it takes at least seventy-two hours of fasting to significantly lower your metabolism.

Can I exercise when fasting?

You can exercise on fasting days, but for the first few weeks, you might want to lower the intensity of your routine until your body gets used to the calorie restriction. Studies have actually shown that you can burn more stored fat when exercising during a fast, so include an aerobic element in your workout to take advantage of that fact.

Can I still have a glass of wine on fasting days?

You can have any kind of alcohol on fasting days, but it's not really a great choice from a calorie perspective. If you want to have a beverage, wine is not the worst selection because it only has about 120 calories per glass, but stay away from sugary drinks if possible. Also, drinking alcohol on a relatively empty stomach can create issues, including increased sensitivity to alcohol effects and the urge to snack.

Do I have to count calories on non-fasting days?

You can eat anything you want on days you're not fasting, but in order to maximize the benefits of fasting, it's a good idea to follow a healthy diet that limits saturated fats, processed foods, and sugar.

MAKING THE TRANSITION

The idea of deliberately depriving yourself of food can be a strange one for many people. Eating is a necessity, and fasting seems somehow unnatural. Once you make the decision to try the 5:2 Diet, it can be hard to shift from your current eating habits to the plan. Here are some strategies you can use to make the transition to the 5:2 Diet easier:

- **Take fasting one day at a time.** Things often look insurmountable when you try to visualize the big picture rather than achievable steps. Fasting every week for the rest of your life might seem overwhelming, but you can certainly do one day. Get through your first day and then move on to the next, and soon your first month of the 5:2 plan will be under your belt.
- **Keep a food journal.** Try to write down everything you eat for at least the first month, both fasting and non-fasting days, so you know exactly

what you're consuming. This could be important if you find yourself unable to drop any weight—if you look at your journal, you can see how many calories you've consumed in the entire week. You might have to adjust your non-fasting days if you find the calorie count is too high to support weight loss.

- **Eat healthfully on non-fasting days.** One of the most attractive features of the 5:2 Diet is that you can eat anything you want on your non-fasting days. However, gorging on pizza, ice cream, and fried chicken will not move you any closer to your health or weight loss goals. You still need to watch what you eat and portion sizes. This is not to say that you can't have a slice of pizza or a piece of chocolate cake, but those food options should be a treat.
- **Keep busy.** Anyone who has forgotten to eat because they were swamped at work or with errands knows the value of staying busy when trying to fast. You won't have time to dwell on food if your schedule is packed, and the day will fly by. For most people, the weekends aren't great fasting days because these are times to relax with family or friends and eat.
- **Enjoy your fasting days.** Fasting will probably be a new experience, so try to listen to your body and enjoy the sensations and changes that occur. You should feel an empowering clarity of thought and lightness of body while fasting. You may not realize that even going twenty-four hours without significant amounts of food can reduce that full, bloated sensation that accompanies eating certain products. Your body will feel lighter and you'll appreciate the food you're eating.

THE FIRST MONTH: WHAT TO EXPECT

The hardest part of starting a new lifestyle is often not knowing what to expect as you go forward. Fasting in particular can be kind of scary because most people like to eat and have never tried to significantly restrict their food intake. Here is what you might experience in the first month of fasting:

- Fasting will test your will power at some point because people are conditioned to eat every few hours rather than going hours without food. You will find it difficult, especially during social situations, not to follow your usual routine.

- You will probably experience loud stomach rumblings, irritability, hunger cravings, and an upset stomach on fasting days and digestion issues on the following days.
- You will lose some weight depending on what you eat on non-fasting days and whether you exercise. To sustain your weight loss, you will need to address any emotional or social triggers that make you overeat.
- You might discover that you eat more junk than you realized as you experience cravings for those foods on fasting days.
- Hunger is not a sensation that continues indefinitely, but rather comes in waves and then recedes.
- Fasting does not make you extra hungry on the following days, so don't worry that you will eat uncontrollably.
- You could feel very tired initially, especially in the afternoon, but that sensation will go away.
- During the first month, you might have trouble sleeping on the evening between your fasting day and regular day because you're hungry.
- You should feel clearer mentally.

FOODS TO AVOID, FOODS TO ENJOY

Your personal food preferences will determine what you eat on the 5:2 Diet, but there are some items that work well on fasting and non-fasting days. This is definitely not a comprehensive list, so feel free to add items that you like, particularly in the fruit and vegetable category. There are foods in the "allowed" list that should be used sparingly because they're higher in fat or calories, such as dairy, nuts, and dried fruit.

Foods to avoid (or limit) include:

- Alcohol
- Butter
- Fatty meats or chicken with skin
- Foods high on the glycemic index
- Fruit juices
- Full-fat milks, cheeses, and other dairy products
- Sugary foods

Foods to enjoy include:

- Vegetables and fruit: Apples (unsweetened applesauce), apricots, bananas, beets, bell peppers, berries (fresh and frozen), broccoli (fresh and frozen), carrots, cauliflower (fresh and frozen), celeriac, celery, cherries, corn (fresh, canned, and frozen), cucumbers, eggplant, garlic, grapefruit, grapes, green beans (fresh and canned), green onion, herbs (fresh and dried), jicama, kiwi, lemons, lettuces, limes, mangoes, melons, mushrooms, onions, oranges, papaya, parsnip, peaches (fresh and canned), pears, pineapple (fresh and canned), plums, potatoes, spinach (fresh and frozen), squash, sweet potatoes, tomatoes (fresh and canned), zucchini
- Protein: Beef (lean), black beans (dried and canned), chicken breast (fresh and frozen skinless), chicken sausage (lean), chickpeas (canned), crab, fish (fresh and frozen—all varieties), ground beef (extra lean), ground chicken (extra lean), ground turkey (extra lean), kidney beans (canned), lentils (dried and canned), navy beans (dried and canned), pinto beans (dried and canned), pork tenderloin, scallops (fresh and frozen), shrimp (fresh and frozen), split peas (dried), turkey breast (boneless, skinless), turkey sausage (lean)
- Grains and breads: Bagels (whole wheat), barley, bread (whole wheat), bulgur, couscous, English muffins (whole wheat), hamburger buns (whole wheat), oats (plain and steel cut), pasta (whole grain), pita bread (whole wheat), quinoa, rice, tortillas (corn and multigrain), wild rice
- Dairy (in moderation): Cheeses (low fat or nonfat), cottage cheese (low fat or nonfat), cream cheese (nonfat), eggs, egg substitute, egg whites, evaporated milk (low fat or skim), milk (skim or 1 percent), sour cream (nonfat), yogurt (nonfat)
- Nuts and seeds (in moderation): Almonds, chia seeds, coconut (unsweetened), flaxseed, hemp seeds, nut butters, peanut butter (natural), pecans, pistachios, pumpkin seeds, sesame seeds, sunflower seeds
- Oils (in moderation): Canola oil, canola oil cooking spray, olive oil, olive oil cooking spray
- Pantry: Agave nectar, brown rice syrup, crisp breads, Dijon mustard, dill pickles, horseradish, hot sauce, maple syrup, miso soup, roasted red bell peppers, salsa, stock (beef, chicken, and vegetable), tamari sauce, vinegar (cider and rice)

KITCHEN TOOLS AND EQUIPMENT

Your kitchen really won't change that much when you're following the 5:2 Diet because you'll still be going about your usual routine for five days out of seven. One effect of the 5:2 plan is that you'll become very aware of your food and the cooking techniques that work best for low-calorie recipes. You obviously don't need anything beyond a few basic tools to make most recipes, but here are some items that will make food preparation and the cooking process easier:

- Real chef knives: It cannot be stated enough how important sharp, well-balanced knives are for the preparation of even basic food. Invest in a selection of knives if it's in your budget; good-quality professional knives will last you a lifetime if you sharpen and clean them properly.
- Other handy tools: Some tools that are very handy for prep work and will save you time are a good peeler, garlic press, grater, and zester.
- Food scale: When every calorie counts, it's important to be able to weigh your food accurately, especially meats. Try to get a digital scale so that you can measure precisely.
- Nonstick cookware: This is crucial for low-calorie cooking because you'll want to use little to no oil to brown or sauté your food. You also might consider a good old-fashioned seasoned cast-iron skillet for cooking.
- Cutting boards: Many people don't consider how handy a nice, large cutting board is until they need one. Choose one that is of good quality, and if you prefer wood boards, make sure they're treated to resist bacteria and rot.
- Food processor, blender, and immersion blender: You probably can survive in the kitchen without these pieces of equipment, but they're wonderful for creating smoothies, soups, and mounds of chopped vegetables or fruit.
- Stainless steel bowls: A nice set of nested bowls will never go to waste in any kitchen because there is always whipping, mixing, and tossing to be done. Stainless steel is the best material because it doesn't rust, stain, or dent.

5:2 DIET COOKING AND PREPARATION TIPS

The strategy on fasting days revolves around not adding any extra unneeded calories or fat to your dishes. This means you might have to reconsider your cooking techniques. Here are a few strategies and tips to create delicious meals for your fasting days:

- Sauté in nonstick cookware with vegetable broth, water, or a very light coating of olive oil spray.
- Use nonfat or low-fat dairy in your recipes.
- Use unsweetened applesauce and mashed banana instead of butter in cakes, cookies, and other baked goods.
- Try different herbs and spices to create interesting dishes.
- Trim all excess skin and fat from your meats.
- Drain any excess fat from your pan and blot your food with clean paper towels.
- Use lemon or lime to intensify flavor in your recipes.
- Spice up your meals with red pepper flakes, fresh hot peppers, and a couple of spoonfuls of salsa.

HOW TO LOSE WEIGHT ON THE 5:2 DIET

Weight loss is often the foremost motive for 5:2 Diet followers, and many have tried other diets in the quest for a lower number on the scale. Most people have a general knowledge about what is required to produce weight loss, but often the practical day-to-day activities toward that loss are difficult to sustain. Plainly stated, if you eat fewer calories than your body uses, you will lose weight, and the converse is also true. Other factors such as exercise, genetics, and medical issues can come into play with respect to weight loss, but that simple equation is still important.

Standard calorie-restriction diets don't usually work long-term because people feel deprived and can't sustain cutting calories indefinitely. This means going back to their original eating habits and gaining all of the weight back, or even more. The 5:2 Diet is a sustainable long-term weight loss solution because you're not dieting constantly, but you're still getting the fat-burning benefits of calorie restriction. Studies have shown that fasting intermittently has the same weight loss effect (and better) than limiting calories constantly (Harvie 2013).

When you don't eat every day, the body starts to burn fat stores, which creates weight loss because your body still needs all the usual energy. When you fast, the body turns to the glucose in the blood, and when the body has used all of the glucose and stored glucose, it breaks down stored fat for energy. This process produces weight loss without slowing the metabolism like full-time calorie-restriction diets. Your body will burn fat at its usual rate or higher when you fast intermittently (Kraemer 2002).

A nice side effect of the weight loss is detoxification: Toxins from environmental factors and food are often stored in the fat of the body, so when you start to burn it, the toxins are also flushed out. When you're fasting, your body actually has time to detoxify because the organs involved in the process, such as the liver and kidneys, get to rest from constantly processing food. Make sure you drink at least eight glasses of water per day to expedite the process.

The 5:2 Diet should produce steady weight loss because two fasting days per week creates an average calorie deficit of 3,500 in the weekly calorie total. Cutting 3,500 calories equals losing one pound of fat.

So what should you do if your diet efforts plateau or you have no new weight loss after a month of following the 5:2 Diet?

- Figure out exactly what you're eating in the week, including non-fast days. If you're consuming too many calories when not fasting, you won't lose weight, so adjust your diet to produce a calorie deficit of at least 3,500 calories per week.
- Try alternate-day fasting for a few weeks instead of just two days per week. This means fasting every other day and should not be attempted without consulting your primary health-care provider.
- Ramp up your exercise program or add more activities that burn calories. Even walking about 10,000 steps per day can burn 2,100 calories a week, so ditch your car to do your errands and get to work, if possible.
- Shock your body with some workout changes to get yourself out of a rut. If you like to jog, change to swimming a few laps instead, or add some circuit training to your weight-training routine. Your body will react by burning more calories.
- Consult with your family doctor to make sure you have no underlying medical problem that prevents weight loss, such as polycystic ovary syndrome or thyroid issues.

EXERCISE AND THE 5:2 DIET

Part of the appeal of the 5:2 Diet is the fact that it's very flexible, and this extends to exercise. In the first few months of the 5:2 Diet, it's important to read your body during fasting days and not overdo your workouts. You can experience some fatigue due to lack of sleep and getting used to fewer calories. If you're a trained athlete or just someone who follows an extensive exercise routine, there might be no real change in your energy or performance. If you don't exercise at all, make sure you start off slowly and work up to a more active lifestyle. It's important to include some sort of exercise in your life to remain healthy and lose weight, if that is your goal.

Fasting and exercise is a very good combination for burning fat. Studies have shown that fasting can create a rise in the level of human growth hormone (HGH) in your system. This surge of HGH will direct the body to burn more fat instead of breaking down muscles, so exercising first thing on your fast days without eating beforehand can accelerate weight loss. Make sure you drink water before and during your workout, though, because water is crucial for many processes in the body. Also, time your first meal, which should include both protein and complex carbohydrates, about 30 minutes after you exercise, especially following a more intense session.

Exercise during a fasting day doesn't have to include huge weights or miles logged on a track—it can be anything that gets your body moving. Some great exercise options for fasting days include:

- Boxing
- Dancing
- Gardening
- Housework
- Martial arts
- Playing with your kids or dog
- Shoveling snow
- Swimming
- Team sports
- Walking
- Walking stairs
- Yoga or Pilates

TEN STEPS FOR 5:2 DIET SUCCESS

Starting a new diet can be exciting and a little scary, so it's important to begin the process with a strategy in mind. Here are ten easy-to-follow steps to guide you to 5:2 Diet success.

1. **Try to eat only when you're hungry.** The way you space your meals on fasting days will be entirely up to you and will depend on schedule, physical need, and habit. If you have a routine built around having a cup of coffee and reading the paper in the morning, you might want to continue that activity. However, if you're not hungry in the morning, then skip breakfast and don't eat until your body signals that it is ready.

2. **Don't forget to exercise.** It's obvious that exercise is crucial if you want to lose body fat and get healthier. So if you're a couch potato, start incorporating some movement into your day, and if you already have an exercise schedule, continue it. The body is made to run, walk, stretch, lift, twist, and jump, so enjoy life by being active.

3. **Fill your plate with vegetables and fruit.** You can pile several cups of raw or steamed produce on a dinner plate to the point where you can barely see the edges and you still might only have 150 calories. Produce is low in calories, cholesterol, sodium, and, for the most part, fat. It's absolutely packed with energy, fiber, and nutrients—and it's delicious.

4. **Save your calories for food.** When you're thirsty on your fasting days, it's best to drink water. You can also drink black coffee and herbal teas when fasting. The beverages you need to stay away from are full-fat milk and fruit juices because they're high in calories. Having a small glass of orange juice can take up about a third of your calorie allotment. It's better to eat your calories in whole, filling foods than drink them in a glass.

5. **Get adequate sleep.** Many people underestimate the value of getting enough sleep when it comes to health and weight loss. Sleep is crucial when fasting because you might already feel a bit fatigued from calorie restriction, and adding tiredness from lack of rest will sabotage your success. Being tired often makes people reach for food in an effort to perk themselves up. Studies have also linked too little sleep with weight gain or failure to lose weight because the metabolism and hormones don't work effectively with too little sleep.

6. **Stay positive.** Everyone reacts differently to eating plans, so don't despair if you don't drop weight quickly or your health doesn't improve immediately. If you need to lose weight, consider the fact that it probably took years to gain that weight, so have the patience to see it go. It's an incredibly positive step to start the 5:2 Diet, so continue to be upbeat and optimistic.

7. **Plan ahead.** One of the main reasons people aren't successful when making food-related lifestyle changes is because they fall back into old eating habits. If you know you're usually exhausted after work and never cook dinner, don't assume because you're fasting that you'll suddenly be flitting around your kitchen joyfully chopping, sautéing, and garnishing. You'll most likely want to reach for something already prepared. So make sure there is something to reach for in your fridge or pantry. Have low-calorie snacks, soups, fruit, cut-up veggies, and a premixed salad ready to go.

8. **Eat on your fasting days.** This might sound like the wrong advice, but you should always eat enough food so that you just make your allotment of calories. When you first begin fasting, five hundred or six hundred calories won't seem like much, but you will soon feel empowered, which might lead you to take it too far. Don't overdo the fasting in an attempt to get quicker results. This diet is meant to be long-term, not the means to get back into your pants from your "skinny" days.

9. **Eat slowly and enjoy your meals.** Eating should never be a race, except if you're at a county fair with a heaping plate of hot dogs in front of you and several other competitors seated at the same table. Savor your food and share your meals with other people whenever possible. One of the best things about fasting is that you learn to eliminate mindless eating on the run. Also, it takes the brain some time to realize you are full, so if you eat slowly, you will feel more satisfied.

10. **Get support.** Find a 5:2 Diet buddy if possible to make the process easier. Sharing the hard moments and successes with someone who is also on the plan can make an incredible difference in your motivation. Your support buddy doesn't necessarily have to be someone you see regularly. There are wonderful communities on 5:2 websites that can offer advice and encouragement to newbie fasters.

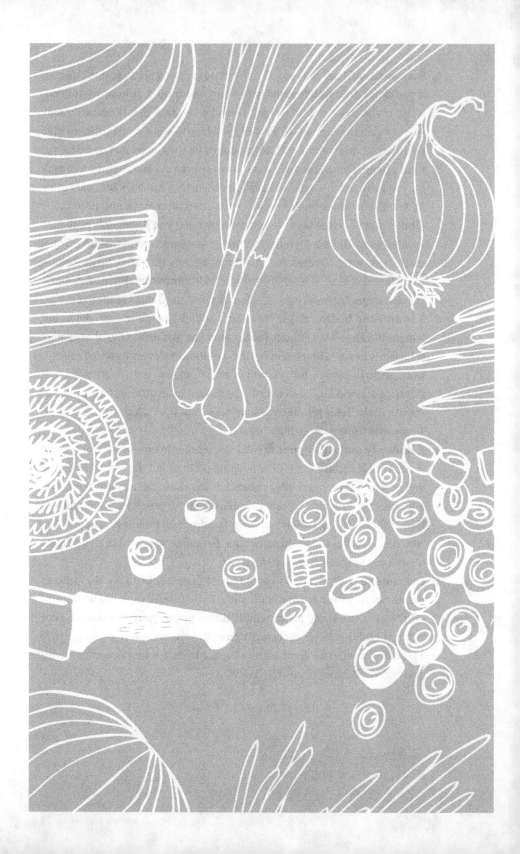

CHAPTER THREE

A Month of Fasting-Day Meal Plans

This meal plan is a tool to help you jump right into the 5:2 Diet for at least a month without having to plan out your fast days yourself. One of the biggest concerns people have when beginning a fasting diet is deciding what they're going to eat and feeling overwhelmed by the process of counting calories. This plan isn't meant to be followed rigidly—the 5:2 Diet is all about flexibility—but rather to be considered a guideline for the days you fast.

TIPS FOR NON-FASTING DAYS

There are no rules in the 5:2 Diet about what you can or cannot eat on your non-fasting days, but there is a bit of gentle advice concerning strategies you can follow in order to get the most benefits from the diet. On your non-fasting days, you might want to:

- Not refer to the days as "feast" days so you won't feel like you have to binge-eat to live up to the label!
- Keep within a 2,000-calorie range if you are a woman and a 2,600 range if you are a man.
- Still try to follow a healthy, nutrient-packed diet rather than consuming saturated fats, sugar, and processed foods, especially if you're trying to lose weight.
- Use these non-fasting days for social events and special occasions that include meals out or special treats like double chocolate cake.
- Ramp up your workout because you have a good supply of calories to fuel your physical efforts.
- Enjoy your food, including your favorite meals and treats.

HOW TO USE THE FASTING-DAY MEAL PLANS

Each fasting-day meal plan that follows is set up as three meals per day, but you can arrange your day in any configuration as long as your calories stay below the allotted number for your gender. Each meal in the plan has the number of calories listed beside it, so you can swap the meals around if you want a different breakfast or have leftovers from the day before to eat for lunch. You can also substitute recipes from the book for the meal plan as long as they have a similar calorie count. The most important part of the fasting-day meal plans is to enjoy your food.

EIGHT FASTING-DAY MEAL PLANS

These eight meal plans add up to one month's worth of fasting days. They are not to be done consecutively, but to be used as part of the 5:2 Diet—five regular eating days interspersed with two (nonconsecutive) fasting days.

* Indicates a recipe in this book

FASTING DAY #1
Daily total: 485 calories

Note: For 600 calories per day, add 1 serving Crunchy Mozzarella Nuggets* as a snack (91 calories).

Breakfast
Yogurt berry parfait (138 calories)
- 3 ounces plain nonfat Greek yogurt
- ½ cup sliced strawberries
- 1 tablespoon low-calorie granola

Lunch
Miso soup (65 calories)
- 3 cups water
- 2 tablespoons miso paste
- 10 snow peas, julienned
- 3 whole bok choy, chopped
- ½ green onion, thinly sliced
- ¼ red bell pepper, julienned
- ¼ cup shredded carrot

Snack

1 cup diced watermelon (50 calories)

Dinner

Prosciutto-Wrapped Chicken* (232 calories) and 1 cup broccoli florets, steamed

FASTING DAY #2
Daily total: 498 calories

Note: For 600 calories per day, add 1 cup baked diced butternut squash (80 calories).

Breakfast

Green Tea, Ginger, and Melon Smoothie* (103 calories)

Lunch

Sausage, Spinach, and White Bean Stew* (261 calories)

Dinner

Baked lemon fish (134 calories)

- 3 ounces salmon fillet
- Squeeze of fresh lemon juice
- Sea salt and freshly ground pepper
- Olive oil cooking spray
- 1 cup loosely packed baby spinach
- 1 teaspoon fat-free balsamic salad dressing

FASTING DAY #3
Daily total: 495 calories

Note: For 600 calories per day, add 1 slice low-calorie whole-wheat bread to lunch, and a tangerine as a snack (100 calories).

Breakfast

Cream of Wheat (161 calories)

- 1 single-serve package Cream of Wheat, cooked with water
- 2 tablespoons nonfat milk
- 1 tablespoon dried cranberries
- 1 teaspoon maple syrup

Lunch

Spicy Tomato Soup* (103 calories)

Dinner

Breaded Chicken Thighs with Lemon and Garlic* (231 calories) and ½ baked sweet potato topped with 1 teaspoon fat-free sour cream and ½ green onion, chopped

FASTING DAY #4
Daily total: 489 calories

Note: For 600 calories per day, add 1 ounce tuna to lunch, and 1 cup blueberries as a snack (110 calories).

Breakfast

Egg White Scramble with Fresh Veggies* (105 calories)

Lunch

Open-faced tuna sandwich with salad (189 calories)
- 1 ounce water-packed tuna
- 1 slice low-calorie multigrain bread
- 2 cups mixed salad greens
- ½ plum tomato, chopped
- ¼ English cucumber, peeled, seeded, and chopped
- ½ cup grated carrot
- Squeeze of fresh lemon juice

Dinner

Rosemary-Garlic Pork Tenderloin* (197 calories) and 2 cups cauliflower florets, steamed

FASTING DAY #5
Daily total: 490 calories

Note: For 600 calories per day, add 3 ounces extra-lean ham to lunch (91 calories).

Breakfast

Scrambled egg whites with tomato (122 calories)
- 3 egg whites
- 5 cherry tomatoes, halved
- 1 tablespoon chopped red onion
- ½ low-calorie English muffin

Lunch
Citrus Salad over Mixed Greens* (60 calories)

Dinner
Turkey Burgers with Sautéed Teriyaki Onions* (308 calories) and 1 large carrot, peeled and cut into sticks

FASTING DAY #6
Daily total: 500 calories

Note: For 600 calories per day, add 1 slice pumpernickel bread to lunch, and a small plum for a snack (95 calories).

Breakfast
Ricotta Toasts with Fresh Fruit* (220 calories)

Lunch
½ red grapefruit with low-calorie sweetener (40 calories)

Dinner
Spicy Baked Tilapia* (240 calories) and 1 cup steamed spinach with squeeze of fresh lemon juice

FASTING DAY #7
Daily total: 493 calories

Note: For 600 calories per day, add ½ plain reduced-calorie bagel with 1 ounce fat-free cream cheese to breakfast (100 calories).

Breakfast
Fresh fruit salad (177 calories)
- ½ large banana, sliced
- ½ mango, peeled, seeded, and chopped
- 1 cup strawberries, sliced

Lunch
Tom Yum Soup* (158 calories)

Dinner
Lemon-Garlic Shrimp* (164 calories) and ½ cup bean sprouts, ½ cup shredded carrot, and 6 snow peas, halved

FASTING DAY #8
Daily total: 491 calories

Note: For 600 calories per day, add 1 serving Cinnamon-Sugar Crisps* as a snack (89 calories).

Breakfast
Strawberry smoothie (103 calories)
- 1 ounce nonfat Greek yogurt
- ½ cup nonfat milk
- ¼ banana, sliced
- 5 medium strawberries, sliced

Lunch
Egg White and Avocado Salad* (179 calories)

Dinner
Grilled steak with butternut squash and green beans (209 calories)
- 3 ounces lean steak (grilled), seasoned
- Sea salt and freshly ground pepper
- 1/2 cup diced butternut squash, steamed or blanched
- 1/2 cup green beans, steamed or blanched

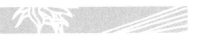

PART TWO

Recipes for Fasting Days

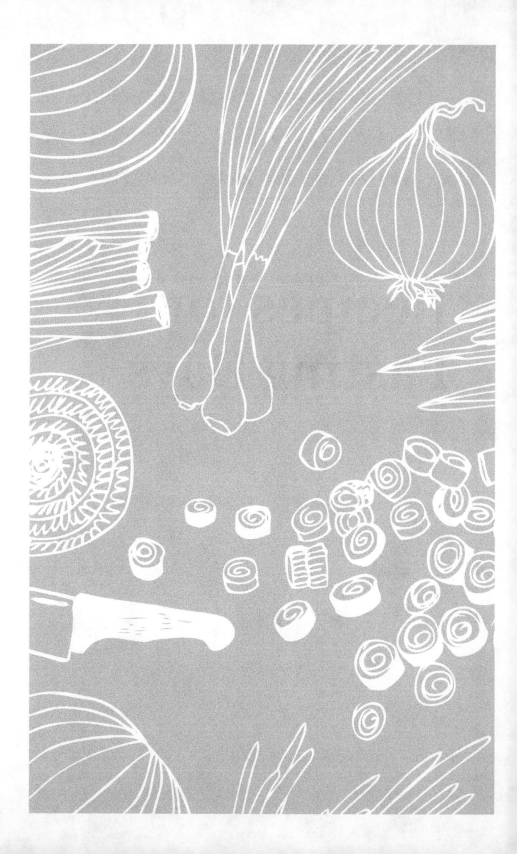

CHAPTER FOUR

Breakfast

Green Tea, Ginger, and Melon Smoothie

SERVES 4

▶ 103 CALORIES PER SERVING
▶ TOTAL PREPARATION TIME: 3 HOURS

Green tea is a nutritional superstar: People who drink it regularly have a lower risk for heart disease and lower cholesterol and blood pressure. If you don't want it hot, this refreshing smoothie is a fun way to get the benefits of green tea. This recipe has a long preparation time, but almost all of it is freezing the tea.

1½ CUPS PLUS 3 TABLESPOONS WATER
2 BAGS GREEN TEA
2 TABLESPOONS SUGAR
1-INCH PIECE OF GINGER, PEELED AND THINLY SLICED
3 CUPS CHOPPED HONEYDEW MELON
ONE 12-OUNCE CAN GINGER ALE
¼ CUP FRESH LEMON JUICE
¼ CUP FRESH MINT LEAVES

1. In a medium saucepan, bring 1½ cups water to a simmer. Remove from heat, add tea bags, and let steep 5 minutes. Remove tea bags and let tea cool to room temperature.

2. In a small saucepan over medium heat, bring 3 tablespoons water, sugar, and ginger to a simmer. Cook, stirring, until sugar dissolves, about 2 minutes. Remove from heat and let cool; discard ginger. Stir ginger syrup into the tea. Pour into ice cube trays and freeze until solid, about 2 hours. Also freeze the chopped melon until solid, about 2 hours.

3. In a blender, combine half of iced tea cubes, half of frozen melon, half the can of ginger ale, half the lemon juice, and half the mint. Purée until smooth and divide between 2 glasses. Repeat with remaining ingredients.

Mixed Berry Smoothie

SERVES 3

▶ 139 CALORIES PER SERVING
▶ TOTAL PREPARATION TIME: 5 MINUTES

This is what most people think of when they hear the word "smoothie." It also couldn't be easier to prepare since it uses frozen berries, which have been shown to pack just as much nutritional punch as fresh ones since they're frozen at their ripest.

1¼ CUPS ORANGE JUICE

1 BANANA

1¼ CUPS FROZEN MIXED BERRIES (RASPBERRIES, BLACKBERRIES, BLUEBERRIES, AND STRAWBERRIES)

½ CUP PLAIN LOW-FAT YOGURT

1 TABLESPOON SUGAR

In a blender, combine all ingredients. Cover and blend until creamy. Serve immediately.

Oatmeal with Berries and Hazelnuts

SERVES 2

▶ 158 CALORIES PER SERVING
▶ TOTAL PREPARATION TIME: 20 MINUTES

Oatmeal is a whole grain, meaning it can lower blood pressure and reduce your risk for diabetes. Unfortunately, the stuff that comes in packets can have lots of sugar and artificial ingredients. Make it yourself and you will know exactly what you're putting into your body.

⅓ CUP QUICK-COOKING OATMEAL
1½ TABLESPOONS COARSELY CHOPPED HAZELNUTS, TOASTED
2 TABLESPOONS GRANOLA WITH RAISINS
PINCH OF SALT
⅓ CUP HOT WATER
1 TABLESPOON HONEY
4 STRAWBERRIES, SLICED
8 RASPBERRIES
2 TEASPOONS SUGAR
LOW-FAT GREEK YOGURT FOR TOPPING

1. In a small bowl, mix together oatmeal, hazelnuts, granola, and salt. Pour hot water and honey over mixture, stir, and set aside to soak for 12 to 15 minutes.

2. In another small bowl, combine strawberries, raspberries, and sugar. Allow to sit while oats are soaking. When ready, divide oats between 2 bowls, top with berries, and stir. Serve with a dollop of yogurt on top.

Apple-Hazelnut Oatmeal

SERVES 4

▶ 387 CALORIES PER SERVING

▶ TOTAL PREPARATION TIME: 30 MINUTES

Oatmeal is already heart healthy, but this version gets an extra boost from the addition of flaxseed. Flaxseed has been shown to lower bad cholesterol and raise good cholesterol, and some studies have shown that it can help fight diabetes, cancer, and stroke. You can find it preground in the grain aisle.

¼ CUP WHOLE HAZELNUTS

3 CUPS NONFAT MILK

1½ CUPS REGULAR OATS

1 GRANNY SMITH APPLE, CORED AND DICED

⅓ CUP GROUND FLAXSEED

½ TEASPOON GROUND CINNAMON

¼ TEASPOON SALT

½ TEASPOON VANILLA EXTRACT

3 TABLESPOONS PACKED BROWN SUGAR

3 TABLESPOONS SLIVERED ALMONDS

1. Preheat oven to 350°F.

2. Place hazelnuts on a baking sheet. Bake for 15 minutes, stirring once halfway through. Place toasted nuts on a towel, roll up, and rub off skins. Finely chop nuts and set aside.

3. In a medium saucepan, combine milk, oats, apple, flaxseed, cinnamon, and salt. Bring to a boil over medium heat and stir in vanilla. Cover, reduce heat to low, and simmer 5 minutes or until thick. Sprinkle with hazelnuts, brown sugar, and almonds, and serve immediately.

Porridge with Raisins and Cinnamon

SERVES 4

▶ 491 CALORIES PER SERVING

▶ TOTAL PREPARATION TIME: 20 MINUTES

Porridge is any hot cereal cooked in boiling milk or water (or both). This version gets its flavor from cinnamon, raisins, and vanilla. Don't worry about the fact that you're adding raw eggs to it—the hot cereal cooks them completely.

3 CUPS WATER

1 CUP POWDERED MILK

1½ CUPS ROLLED OATS

½ TEASPOON GROUND CINNAMON

½ CUP RAISINS

½ TEASPOON VANILLA EXTRACT

3 EGGS

4 TEASPOONS UNSALTED BUTTER

1 CUP NONFAT MILK

2 TABLESPOONS HONEY

1. Bring water to a boil in a large saucepan. In a medium bowl, combine powdered milk, oats, and cinnamon. Stir into boiling water, return to a boil, and reduce heat and simmer for 5 to 10 minutes or until it reaches your desired thickness.

2. Remove from heat and mix in raisins and vanilla. Beat in the eggs one at a time. Top with butter, milk, and honey.

Baked Eggs in Tomato Sauce

SERVES 4

▶ 263 CALORIES PER SERVING
▶ TOTAL PREPARATION TIME: 40 MINUTES

Roasting the tomatoes first gives the sauce a smoky, richer flavor. If you only want to make one serving at a time, make the entire batch of sauce, then pour a quarter of it into a ramekin and top with 2 eggs and some cheese. The sauce will keep in the refrigerator so you can make the rest later in the week.

1½ POUNDS PLUM TOMATOES, HALVED LENGTHWISE
1 GARLIC CLOVE, SMASHED
2 TABLESPOONS OLIVE OIL
SALT AND FRESHLY GROUND PEPPER
1 TEASPOON CHOPPED FRESH OREGANO
8 EGGS
2 TABLESPOONS GRATED PARMESAN CHEESE

1. Preheat oven to 400°F.

2. In a roasting pan, mix together tomatoes, garlic, and oil. Season with salt and pepper. Arrange tomatoes cut side up and roast for 15 minutes. Turn tomatoes over and roast 20 minutes or until soft. Let tomatoes cool slightly, then scrape everything from the pan into a blender. Purée and add oregano.

3. Place 4 shallow ovenproof bowls on a baking sheet. Pour tomato sauce through a strainer into the bowls. Crack 2 eggs into each bowl and season with salt and pepper. Sprinkle eggs with cheese and bake for 15 minutes or until whites are set.

Quinoa Egg Bake with Spinach

SERVES 4

▶ 390 CALORIES PER SERVING
▶ TOTAL PREPARATION TIME: 65 MINUTES

Quinoa is a grain, but it's also packed with protein and amino acids. Usually you need to cook it on its own, but because this dish is baked in the oven, you can use it without precooking it. Make sure not to skip the rinsing step—quinoa can have a bitter coating that needs to be washed off before using.

1 TEASPOON UNSALTED BUTTER

½ CUP UNCOOKED QUINOA

8 EGGS

1¼ CUPS NONFAT MILK

1 TABLESPOON CHOPPED GARLIC

1 TEASPOON CHOPPED FRESH THYME

½ TEASPOON SALT

½ TEASPOON FRESHLY GROUND PEPPER

2 CUPS PACKED BABY SPINACH, CHOPPED

1 CUP SHREDDED PARMESAN CHEESE

1. Preheat oven to 350°F.

2. Grease an 8-by-8-inch glass baking dish with butter.

3. Place quinoa in a fine mesh strainer and rinse with cold water; drain well.

4. In a large bowl, whisk together eggs, milk, garlic, thyme, salt, pepper, and quinoa. Stir in spinach and pour mixture into baking dish. Cover with foil and shake dish gently to settle quinoa on the bottom.

5. Bake 45 minutes or until eggs are just set. Remove foil, sprinkle top with cheese, return to oven, and bake uncovered 10 to 15 more minutes or until golden brown and crisp. Let cool briefly before slicing and serving.

Egg White Scramble with Fresh Veggies

SERVES 1

▶ 105 CALORIES PER SERVING
▶ TOTAL PREPARATION TIME: 5 MINUTES

For mornings when you need to eat something and run out the door, this deconstructed omelet is perfect. Switch up the vegetables if you don't like green pepper or green onion. Tomato, red pepper, and mushrooms would also be delicious.

COOKING SPRAY
½ CUP EGG WHITES
⅓ CUP BABY SPINACH, CHOPPED
1 TABLESPOON FINELY CHOPPED GREEN PEPPER
1 TABLESPOON FINELY CHOPPED GREEN ONION
2 TABLESPOONS REDUCED-FAT SHREDDED MOZZARELLA CHEESE
SALT AND FRESHLY GROUND PEPPER

1. Spray the inside of a large microwave-safe mug with cooking spray.

2. In a small bowl, whisk together egg whites, spinach, pepper, onion, and 1 tablespoon of cheese. Season with salt and pepper. Pour into mug and microwave for 1 minute. Stir and then microwave for 30 more seconds, or until eggs are set. Sprinkle with remaining 1 tablespoon cheese, and enjoy.

Egg Scramble with Smoked Salmon

SERVES 4

▶ 297 CALORIES PER SERVING
▶ TOTAL PREPARATION TIME: 15 MINUTES

Smoked salmon is often paired with a bagel and cream cheese. This twist has the salmon being scrambled in with eggs and then dotted with the cream cheese. Pumpernickel toast takes the place of a bagel here for a lighter dish.

6 EGGS
4 EGG WHITES
1 TEASPOON CANOLA OIL
⅓ CUP SLICED GREEN ONIONS
4 OUNCES SMOKED SALMON, CUT INTO ½-INCH PIECES
2 OUNCES REDUCED-FAT CREAM CHEESE, CUT INTO 12 PIECES
¼ TEASPOON FRESHLY GROUND PEPPER
4 SLICES PUMPERNICKEL BREAD, TOASTED

1. In a medium bowl, whisk together eggs and egg whites.

2. Heat a medium nonstick skillet over medium-high heat. Pour oil into pan and swirl to coat. Add green onions and sauté until tender, about 2 minutes. Add eggs and cook until mixture sets on bottom without stirring. Scrape bottom of pan with spatula to break up eggs. Add salmon and cream cheese, and continue stirring occasionally with spatula. When mixture thickens to your liking, remove from stove. Season with pepper and serve with toast.

Frittata with Butternut Squash and Sage

SERVES 4

▶ 360 CALORIES PER SERVING

▶ TOTAL PREPARATION TIME: 45 MINUTES

Sage pairs wonderfully with sweet vegetables like pumpkin and butternut squash. The squash is roasted first, so it caramelizes and adds a nice crispiness to the final dish.

4 CUPS CUBED BUTTERNUT SQUASH

½ RED ONION, CUT INTO THICK SLICES

1 TABLESPOON OLIVE OIL

1 TEASPOON SALT, DIVIDED

½ TEASPOON FRESHLY GROUND PEPPER, DIVIDED

8 EGGS

⅓ CUP WHOLE MILK

2 TABLESPOONS CHOPPED FRESH SAGE

1 CUP GRATED GRUYÈRE CHEESE

1. Preheat oven to 425°F.

2. Place squash and onion in a large ovenproof skillet and toss with oil, ½ teaspoon salt, and ¼ teaspoon pepper. Roast until vegetables are browned and softened, about 25 minutes, stirring once or twice during cooking. Remove from oven and set aside to cool slightly.

3. In a large bowl, whisk together eggs, milk, sage, remaining ½ teaspoon salt, and remaining ¼ teaspoon pepper. Pour into skillet with the squash and return to oven. Cook until eggs are almost set, about 6 minutes. Remove from oven and sprinkle with cheese. Turn on broiler and place skillet under broiler until cheese melts and top of frittata is brown, about 2 minutes. Cut into wedges and serve.

Frittata with Zucchini and Tomatoes

SERVES 4

▶ 183 CALORIES PER SERVING
▶ TOTAL PREPARATION TIME: 20 MINUTES

A frittata is like a quiche, but without the buttery pie crust. As a result, it's lower in fat and calories and is a perfect healthy breakfast. Make it early in the week and reheat wedges every morning to save yourself time.

6 EGG WHITES

4 EGGS

½ CUP GRATED ROMANO CHEESE, DIVIDED

1 TABLESPOON MINCED FRESH SAGE

½ TEASPOON SALT

¼ TEASPOON FRESHLY GROUND PEPPER

COOKING SPRAY

1 TEASPOON OLIVE OIL

1 ZUCCHINI, SLICED

2 GREEN ONIONS, SLICED

2 PLUM TOMATOES, THINLY SLICED

1. In a large bowl, whisk together egg whites, eggs, ¼ cup Romano cheese, sage, salt, and pepper.

2. Coat a medium ovenproof skillet with cooking spray. Place over medium heat and heat oil. Sauté zucchini and green onions for 2 minutes. Add egg mixture, cover, and cook for 4 to 6 minutes or until eggs are nearly set.

3. Take cover off and top with tomato slices and remaining ¼ cup cheese. Turn on broiler and broil frittata 3 to 4 inches from the heat for 2 to 3 minutes or until eggs are completely set. Let stand for 5 minutes and cut into wedges.

Breakfast Burrito

SERVES 2

▶ 259 CALORIES PER SERVING
▶ TOTAL PREPARATION TIME: 15 MINUTES

This is already a healthy dish, but if you're worried about cholesterol, you can use egg whites instead of eggs and substitute nonfat milk and cheese. While it's called a breakfast burrito, you can turn this into a light dinner by adding a side of black beans and some brown rice.

2 EGGS

1 TABLESPOON 1-PERCENT MILK

1 TEASPOON CHOPPED FRESH CILANTRO

⅛ TEASPOON SALT

DASH OF FRESHLY GROUND PEPPER

COOKING SPRAY

½ TEASPOON UNSALTED BUTTER

TWO 8-INCH FAT-FREE FLOUR TORTILLAS

4 TABLESPOONS REDUCED-FAT SHREDDED CHEDDAR CHEESE

4 TABLESPOONS CHOPPED TOMATO

2 TABLESPOONS JARRED SALSA

1. In a medium bowl, mix together eggs, milk, cilantro, salt, and pepper.

2. Spray a medium nonstick skillet with cooking spray, place over medium heat, and melt butter. Add egg mixture and scramble, stirring with a spatula and pushing the cooked egg toward the center so the uncooked egg can run underneath it around the edges.

3. In a small nonstick skillet, warm tortillas over medium-high heat. Sprinkle 2 tablespoons cheese down the center of each, divide eggs between them, and top with tomato and salsa. Roll up burrito-style and serve.

Migas

SERVES 4

▶ 336 CALORIES PER SERVING
▶ TOTAL PREPARATION TIME: 20 MINUTES

This Tex-Mex breakfast usually combines scrambled eggs with tortilla chips. It is delicious on its own or can be topped with any favorite Mexican ingredients like salsa and avocado. Also feel free to add any vegetables for texture like onion, green pepper, or tomato.

4 TEASPOONS CORN OIL
TWELVE 6-INCH CORN TORTILLAS
6 EGGS, BEATEN
SALT

1. In a large skillet, heat the oil over medium-high heat. Rip corn tortillas into bite-size pieces. Fry them in the skillet, stirring constantly, until they begin to get crispy.

2. Pour the eggs into the skillet with the tortillas, scrambling until eggs are cooked through (push the cooked edges toward the center and allow the uncooked eggs to flow out to the edges). Season with salt and serve immediately.

Breakfast Pizza

SERVES 2

▶ 480 CALORIES PER SERVING
▶ TOTAL PREPARATION TIME: 25 MINUTES

It may sound weird, but breakfast ingredients make a pretty delicious pizza. This recipe calls for scrambled eggs, sausage, cheese, and potatoes, but you can also top it with ham, tomatoes, feta, green peppers, and avocado.

4 TEASPOONS OLIVE OIL
1 RED POTATO, DICED
2 TABLESPOONS WATER
¼ CUP DICED ONION
2 TURKEY BREAKFAST SAUSAGE LINKS, CASINGS REMOVED
2 EGGS, LIGHTLY BEATEN
SALT AND FRESHLY GROUND PEPPER
2 WHOLE-WHEAT PITAS
¼ CUP GRATED CHEDDAR CHEESE
¼ CUP JARRED SALSA

1. In a small saucepan over medium heat, pour 2 teaspoons of the oil. Add potato and water and cover. Cook for 10 to 15 minutes or until potato is tender, stirring often.

2. Meanwhile, in a nonstick skillet over medium heat, heat remaining 2 teaspoons oil. Sauté onion and sausage, breaking sausage up with a fork, until sausage is cooked through. Add eggs, season with salt and pepper, and scramble in pan until just cooked.

3. Top pitas with egg and sausage mixture, and then with potatoes and cheese. Toast in a toaster oven until cheese is melted. Remove and top with salsa.

Ricotta Toasts with Fresh Fruit

SERVES 2

▶ 220 CALORIES PER SERVING
▶ TOTAL PREPARATION TIME: 5 MINUTES

Ricotta is a soft cheese usually found in the dairy aisle near the sour cream. It has a mild, creamy flavor that goes well with sweet fruit. If you don't like pineapple and strawberries, use any other fruit in this breakfast dish.

½ CUP FINELY CHOPPED FRESH PINEAPPLE

4 TABLESPOONS PART-SKIM RICOTTA CHEESE

2 SLICES WHOLE-GRAIN BREAD, TOASTED

4 STRAWBERRIES, SLICED

2 TABLESPOONS CHOPPED WALNUTS

In a small bowl, combine pineapple and ricotta cheese. Spread evenly on toast and top with strawberries and walnuts.

Classic French Toast

SERVES 2

▶ 474 CALORIES PER SERVING
▶ TOTAL PREPARATION TIME: 20 MINUTES

Whole-wheat bread adds fiber to this breakfast favorite. You can also use cinnamon-raisin bread for even more flavor. Add protein to the meal with some sausage or bacon.

2 TABLESPOONS VEGETABLE OIL

2 EGGS

1 TEASPOON GROUND CINNAMON

1 TEASPOON GROUND GINGER

1 TEASPOON GROUND NUTMEG

4 THICK SLICES WHOLE-WHEAT BREAD

½ CUP STRAWBERRIES, SLICED

2 TABLESPOONS HONEY

2 TABLESPOONS POWDERED SUGAR

1. Heat a small nonstick skillet over medium heat. Add 1 tablespoon of the oil to pan and swirl to coat.

2. In a shallow dish, beat together eggs, cinnamon, ginger, and nutmeg. Taking 1 piece of bread at a time, dip both sides into egg mixture. Place 2 pieces in the skillet and cook 3 to 4 minutes or until golden brown on bottom. Flip and cook on other side for 3 to 4 minutes or until done.

3. Add remaining 1 tablespoon oil to pan and repeat with remaining 2 slices of bread.

4. Top French toast with strawberries, honey, and powdered sugar, and serve immediately.

Blueberry Pancakes

SERVES 4

▶ 290 CALORIES PER SERVING
▶ TOTAL PREPARATION TIME: 30 MINUTES

There is something so comforting about a plate of warm blueberry pancakes on a weekend morning. This recipe calls for almond milk, but you can substitute soy milk as long as it's unsweetened. If you don't eat all the pancakes, they can be frozen and reheated.

2 CUPS WHOLE-WHEAT PASTRY FLOUR
2 TEASPOONS BAKING POWDER
1 TEASPOON GROUND CINNAMON
¼ TEASPOON SALT
1 CUP UNSWEETENED ALMOND MILK
½ CUP WATER
2 TABLESPOONS HONEY
1 TEASPOON VANILLA EXTRACT
1¼ CUP FRESH OR FROZEN BLUEBERRIES
COOKING SPRAY

1. In a large bowl, whisk together flour, baking powder, cinnamon, and salt. In a medium bowl, whisk together almond milk, water, honey, and vanilla. Pour liquid ingredients into dry ingredients and stir until mixed. Let batter rest for 10 minutes. Fold blueberries into batter.

2. Take a large nonstick skillet, coat it with cooking spray, and heat it over medium heat until hot. Ladle ¼ cup of the batter at a time onto the skillet and cook 2 minutes or until bottom is golden. Flip and cook 1 to 2 more minutes or until pancakes are cooked through. Repeat with remaining batter. Serve warm.

German Pancakes

SERVES 4

▶ 358 CALORIES PER SERVING

▶ TOTAL PREPARATION TIME: 25 MINUTES

This breakfast favorite is also sometimes called a Dutch baby pancake. It's made in an ovenproof skillet and puffs way up in the pan. It falls when you take it out of the oven, so don't be surprised.

4 EGGS

¼ TEASPOON SALT

1 CUP FLOUR

1 CUP NONFAT MILK

5 TABLESPOONS UNSALTED BUTTER

1 TABLESPOON FRESH LEMON JUICE

2 TABLESPOONS POWDERED SUGAR

1. Preheat oven to 425°F.

2. In a medium bowl, combine eggs, salt, flour, and milk. Melt butter in microwave and pour into a 9-by-13-inch baking pan. Pour batter into pan.

3. Bake for 15 to 20 minutes or until the mixture puffs up. Sprinkle with lemon juice and powdered sugar and serve immediately.

Peanut Butter Pancakes

▶ 436 CALORIES PER SERVING
▶ TOTAL PREPARATION TIME: 15 MINUTES

Peanut butter adds a shot of protein to carb-heavy pancakes. Top with sliced bananas or berries and you won't even miss the butter and maple syrup.

1½ CUPS FLOUR
6 TABLESPOONS SUGAR
2 TEASPOONS BAKING POWDER
¼ TEASPOON SALT
1¼ CUPS NONFAT MILK
¼ CUP CHUNKY PEANUT BUTTER
1 TABLESPOON PEANUT OIL OR VEGETABLE OIL
½ TEASPOON VANILLA EXTRACT
2 EGGS, LIGHTLY BEATEN

1. In a large bowl, mix together flour, sugar, baking powder, and salt. In a medium bowl, stir together milk, peanut butter, oil, vanilla, and eggs. Pour liquid ingredients into dry ingredients and stir until smooth.

2. Heat a nonstick skillet over medium-high heat. Spoon ¼ cup batter at a time onto skillet. When bottom is browned and top begins to bubble, flip pancakes over. Cook until other side is done. Serve warm.

Waffles from Scratch

SERVES 4

▶ 491 CALORIES PER SERVING
▶ TOTAL PREPARATION TIME: 20 MINUTES

Sure, you can buy waffle mix from the grocery store, but why bother when it's so easy to make it yourself? All of the ingredients are items from your pantry, so you can make this without any planning ahead. Beating the egg whites separately makes the waffles light and airy instead of dense.

2 CUPS FLOUR
4 TEASPOONS BAKING POWDER
¼ TEASPOON SALT
1½ CUPS NONFAT MILK
6 TABLESPOONS VEGETABLE OIL
2 EGGS, SEPARATED
COOKING SPRAY

1. Preheat waffle iron.

2. In a large bowl, sift together flour, baking powder, and salt.

3. In a small bowl, stir together milk, oil, and egg yolks. Add to flour mixture and stir until smooth.

4. In a medium bowl, beat egg whites until they form soft peaks. Fold egg whites into batter.

5. When waffle iron is hot, spray with cooking spray. Pour ⅓ cup batter into waffle iron and cook until golden. Repeat with remaining batter. Serve warm.

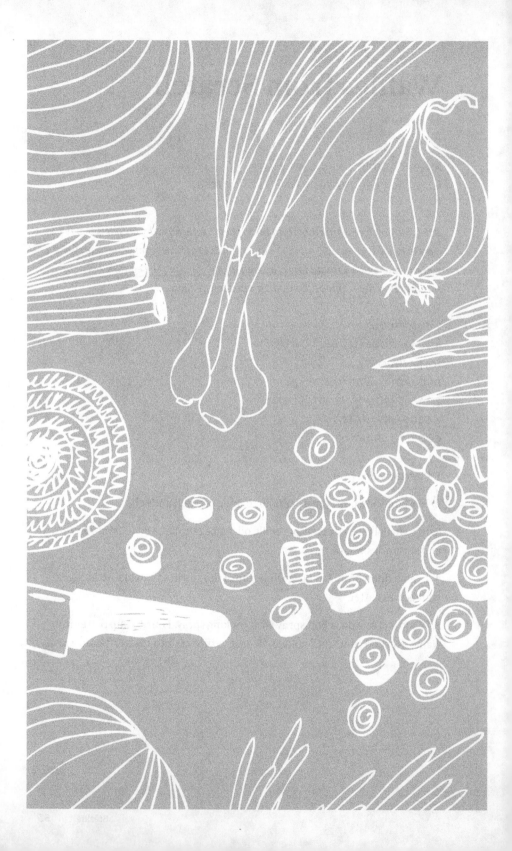

CHAPTER FIVE

Soups and Salads

Spicy Tomato Soup

SERVES 4

▶ 103 CALORIES PER SERVING
▶ TOTAL PREPARATION TIME: 45 MINUTES

Tomatoes are packed with lycopene, a type of antioxidant that is a powerful cancer fighter. They shine in this flavorful soup with a dollop of whipped cream on top that makes it hard to believe it's healthy. The horseradish gives the cream a kick, but you can leave it out if you don't like the strong taste.

1 TABLESPOON UNSALTED BUTTER
½ ONION, DICED
1 CELERY STALK, FINELY CHOPPED
1 GARLIC CLOVE, MINCED
1 TABLESPOON WORCESTERSHIRE SAUCE
ONE 28-OUNCE CAN WHOLE TOMATOES, UNDRAINED
SALT AND FRESHLY GROUND PEPPER
2 TEASPOONS GRATED HORSERADISH
2 TABLESPOONS HEAVY CREAM
1 TABLESPOON CHOPPED FRESH CHIVES

1. In a medium saucepan over medium heat, melt butter. Add onion and celery and cook, stirring, until softened and translucent, about 5 minutes. Add garlic and sauté 1 minute. Add Worcestershire sauce and sauté 1 more minute.

2. While tomatoes are still in the can, cut them into large chunks with kitchen shears. Pour tomatoes and juice into the pan and season with salt and pepper. Bring to a boil over high heat, then reduce to a simmer and cook 20 minutes, stirring occasionally. Remove from heat and stir in 1 teaspoon horseradish. Let cool slightly, then purée in a blender. Strain with a fine mesh sieve and throw out any solids.

3. In a medium bowl, use an electric mixer to whip cream and remaining 1 teaspoon horseradish until it forms stiff peaks. Top soup with horseradish cream and chives and serve immediately.

Italian-Style Tomato Soup with Chickpeas and Pasta

SERVES 4

▶ 425 CALORIES PER SERVING
▶ TOTAL PREPARATION TIME: 26 MINUTES

Enjoy comfort food the way the Romans do with this rustic dish, referred to by Italians as pasta e ceci. *Make the recipe your own, and add red pepper flakes to make it spicy or substitute the chicken broth with vegetable broth to make it a vegetarian dish. If the soup is too thick for your taste, lighten it up with a bit of water.*

3 TABLESPOONS OLIVE OIL
2 CUPS THINLY SLICED YELLOW ONIONS
3 GARLIC CLOVES, CRUSHED
1 TABLESPOON FINELY MINCED FRESH ROSEMARY
ONE 28-OUNCE CAN DICED TOMATOES, UNDRAINED
ONE 15-OUNCE CAN CHICKPEAS, DRAINED
3 CUPS LOW-SODIUM CHICKEN BROTH
SALT AND FRESHLY GROUND PEPPER
1½ CUPS SMALL DRIED PASTA
FRESHLY GRATED PARMESAN CHEESE FOR GARNISHING

In a Dutch oven or large saucepan, heat oil over medium heat. Sauté onion for 7 minutes, until softened, stirring constantly. Add garlic, sauté for 1 minute. Stir in rosemary until well combined. Pour in tomatoes; bring to a boil. Stir in chickpeas and broth; season with salt and pepper and return to a boil. Pour in pasta; cover partially and cook for 10 minutes, until pasta is al dente, stirring occasionally. Divide among bowls and garnish with a sprinkle of Parmesan cheese.

Tom Yum Soup

SERVES 4

▶ 158 CALORIES PER SERVING
▶ TOTAL PREPARATION TIME: 35 MINUTES

Tom Yum is a Thai soup that combines hot and sour flavors. This one gets protein from shrimp, but you can leave them out and substitute vegetable broth for a vegetarian dish.

1 STALK LEMONGRASS, WHITE PART ONLY, CUT INTO 1-INCH PIECES
2¼-INCH-THICK SLICE FRESH GINGER
6 CUPS LOW-SODIUM CHICKEN BROTH
2 JALAPEÑOS, SEEDED, DERIBBED, AND SLICED
THREE 2-INCH STRIPS LIME ZEST
1½ CUPS CHOPPED FRESH PINEAPPLE
1 CUP SLICED SHIITAKE MUSHROOM CAPS
1 TOMATO, CHOPPED
½ RED BELL PEPPER, SEEDED, DERIBBED, AND COARSELY CHOPPED
2 TABLESPOONS FISH SAUCE
1 TEASPOON SUGAR
8 OUNCES SHRIMP, PEELED AND DEVEINED (26 TO 30 COUNT PER POUND)
¼ CUP FRESH LIME JUICE
2 GREEN ONIONS, SLICED
⅓ CUP CHOPPED FRESH CILANTRO

1. Using the broad side of a knife, smash the lemongrass and ginger on a cutting board. Place lemongrass and ginger in a large saucepan and add broth, jalapeños, and lime zest. Bring to a boil over high heat, reduce to a simmer, cover, and cook for 15 minutes. Strain into a bowl and discard solids.

2. Return broth to the pan and add pineapple, mushrooms, tomato, bell pepper, fish sauce, and sugar. Bring to a simmer and cook, uncovered, for 5 minutes. Add shrimp and cook until they are pink and cooked through, 2 to 3 minutes. Remove from heat and stir in lime juice, green onions, and cilantro just before serving.

Spicy Chicken Ginger Soup

SERVES 4

▶ 470 CALORIES PER SERVING
▶ TOTAL PREPARATION TIME: 40 MINUTES

This cayenne-spiked spicy soup will help take the bite out of a cold, blustery day. Finishing the fragrant dish off with a squeeze of lime gives the gingery broth a spirited sour kick.

1 TABLESPOON OLIVE OIL
1 ONION, THINLY SLICED
½ CUP SLICED SHIITAKE MUSHROOMS
1 GARLIC CLOVE, FINELY MINCED
1-INCH PIECE FRESH GINGER, PEELED AND CHOPPED
SALT AND FRESHLY GROUND PEPPER
4 CUPS SHREDDED ROTISSERIE CHICKEN
2 QUARTS LOW-SODIUM CHICKEN BROTH
½ TEASPOON CAYENNE PEPPER
1 CUP PACKED BABY SPINACH
2 GREEN ONIONS, THINLY SLICED
LIME WEDGES (OPTIONAL)

In a large saucepan, heat oil over medium-high heat. Sauté onion and mushrooms for 8 to 10 minutes, until softened, stirring occasionally. Stir in garlic and ginger; sauté for 2 minutes. Season with salt and pepper. Stir in shredded chicken, broth, and cayenne; bring to a boil. Reduce heat and add spinach, and cook until the spinach wilts, 1 to 3 minutes. Divide among bowls and top off with green onions. Serve with lime wedges (if using).

Curried Red Lentil Soup

SERVES 4

▶ 374 CALORIES PER SERVING
▶ TOTAL PREPARATION TIME: 30 MINUTES

Spice up your everyday menu with flavorful curries. If you're trying to reduce how much meat you're eating, red lentils are an efficient source of protein and heart-healthy fiber. One ounce serves up almost 9 grams of protein and 9 grams of dietary fiber.

3 TABLESPOONS CANOLA OIL
2 GARLIC CLOVES, MINCED
2 TABLESPOONS GRATED PEELED FRESH GINGER
8 GREEN ONIONS, SLICED, WHITE AND GREEN PARTS SEPARATED
1 TABLESPOON CURRY POWDER
4 CARROTS, PEELED AND CHOPPED
1 RUSSET POTATO, PEELED AND CHOPPED
1 CUP RED LENTILS
4 CUPS LOW-SODIUM VEGETABLE BROTH
¾ TEASPOON SALT
¼ TEASPOON FRESHLY GROUND PEPPER
LIME WEDGES

In a Dutch oven or large saucepan, heat oil over medium heat. Sauté garlic, ginger, and onion whites for 3 minutes, stirring often. Add curry powder; stir until well combined. Stir in carrots, potato, lentils, broth, salt, and pepper. Bring to a boil; reduce heat and simmer for 15 to 20 minutes, stirring occasionally, until lentils are tender. Divide curry among plates; serve garnished with onion greens and lime wedges.

Sausage, Spinach, and White Bean Stew

SERVES 4

▶ 261 CALORIES PER SERVING
▶ TOTAL PREPARATION TIME: 20 MINUTES

If you're growing tired of your usual proteins, give sweet Italian turkey sausage a try. This recipe combines the seasoned sausage with fiber-filled beans and vitamin-packed spinach to create a hearty, comforting meal.

10 OUNCES SWEET ITALIAN TURKEY SAUSAGE
COOKING SPRAY
1 CUP CHOPPED ONION
2 TEASPOONS MINCED GARLIC
½ CUP WATER
ONE 15-OUNCE CAN CANNELLINI BEANS, RINSED AND DRAINED
ONE 14.5-OUNCE CAN STEWED TOMATOES, UNDRAINED
ONE 14-OUNCE CAN FAT-FREE, LOW-SODIUM CHICKEN BROTH
2 CUPS PACKED BABY SPINACH
2 TEASPOONS CHOPPED FRESH OREGANO
1 TABLESPOON CHOPPED FRESH BASIL
2 TABLESPOONS FRESHLY GRATED ROMANO CHEESE

1. Using kitchen scissors or a paring knife, remove casings from the sausage.

2. Coat a Dutch oven or a large saucepan with cooking spray and heat over medium-high heat. Brown sausage in pan, stirring often to break up and crumble. Mix in onion and garlic; sauté for 2 minutes. Pour in water, beans, tomatoes, and broth; cover and bring to a boil. Uncover and cook for 3 minutes or until thickened. Remove from heat and stir in spinach, oregano, and basil. Top each serving with 1½ teaspoons of cheese.

Classic Beef Chili with Cheddar Cheese

SERVES 4

▶ 427 CALORIES PER SERVING
▶ TOTAL PREPARATION TIME: 40 MINUTES

Whereas many chili recipes call for long simmer times, this one promises a delicious outcome after only 30 minutes. If you would like to knock off some calories from this dish, you can cut out the cheddar cheese, which comes to 57 calories per serving.

2 TABLESPOONS OLIVE OIL
1 ONION, CHOPPED
2 GARLIC CLOVES, MINCED
2 TABLESPOONS CHILI POWDER
1 TEASPOON GROUND CUMIN
2 TEASPOONS GROUND OREGANO
½ TEASPOON CRUSHED RED PEPPER FLAKES
1 POUND LEAN GROUND BEEF
ONE 15-OUNCE CAN TOMATO SAUCE
1 CUP WATER
1 CUP CANNED KIDNEY BEANS
1 CUP CANNED BLACK BEANS
SALT
½ CUP CHOPPED FRESH CILANTRO (OPTIONAL)
HOT PEPPER SAUCE (OPTIONAL)
1 CUP SHREDDED CHEDDAR CHEESE

In a Dutch oven or large saucepan, heat oil over medium heat. Sauté onions and garlic for 5 minutes, stirring frequently. Add chili powder, cumin, oregano, and crushed red pepper; cook for 1 minute, stirring constantly. Stir in ground meat; brown for 3 to 5 minutes. Stir in tomato sauce, water, and beans.

Season with salt and bring to a boil. Reduce heat, cover, and simmer for 30 minutes, stirring often, until sauce is bubbling. Mix in cilantro and hot pepper sauce (if using). Divide chili among four bowls and top each off with 1/4 cup cheddar cheese.

Citrus Salad over Mixed Greens

▶ 60 CALORIES PER SERVING

▶ TOTAL PREPARATION TIME: 10 MINUTES

Citrus fruit shines in the winter, when it can be tough to find produce that's in season. Play around with what you can find in the grocery store—blood oranges and red grapefruit would make a gorgeous version of this salad.

½ GRAPEFRUIT, PEELED

½ ORANGE, PEELED

5 CUPS MIXED GREENS

½ RED ONION, CUT INTO THIN SLICES

1 TABLESPOON CIDER VINEGAR

1½ TEASPOONS FRESH LIME JUICE

1½ TEASPOONS OLIVE OIL

1½ TEASPOONS WATER

⅛ TEASPOON CRUSHED GARLIC

⅛ TEASPOON FRESHLY GROUND PEPPER

⅛ TEASPOON CUMIN

1. Cut grapefruit and orange into bite-size pieces and place in a large bowl. Toss with greens and onion.

2. In a medium bowl, whisk together vinegar, lime juice, oil, water, garlic, pepper, and cumin. Drizzle over salad and toss well.

Egg White and Avocado Salad

SERVES 4

▶ 179 CALORIES PER SERVING
▶ TOTAL PREPARATION TIME: 5 MINUTES

The classic egg salad gets a healthy makeover here by using only the egg whites. Avocado adds the creaminess that the yolks would have, while apple gives the salad a nice crunch. This is served over lettuce, but it also makes a great filling for a sandwich.

6 HARD-BOILED EGG WHITES, CHOPPED
2 TABLESPOONS LIGHT MAYONNAISE
1 GRANNY SMITH APPLE, CORED AND DICED
1 AVOCADO, PEELED AND CHOPPED
2 TABLESPOONS FRESH LEMON JUICE
1 TABLESPOON MINCED FRESH PARSLEY
4 CUPS CHOPPED LETTUCE

In a medium bowl, gently mix together egg whites, mayonnaise, apple, avocado, lemon juice, and parsley. Serve over lettuce.

Tuna and Chickpea Salad with Lemon Vinaigrette

SERVES 4

▶ 298 CALORIES PER SERVING
▶ TOTAL PREPARATION TIME: 65 MINUTES

Cans of tuna are a pantry staple that should not be overlooked. For this recipe, you're asked to use tuna packed in olive oil—be sure to reserve the oil, which will be used to make a tasty vinaigrette. This salad holds up well and will taste even better on the second day, after the flavors have had time to linger together.

1 RED ONION, HALVED AND CUT INTO THIN SLICES
2 GARLIC CLOVES, CRUSHED
3 TABLESPOONS OLIVE OIL
ONE 6- TO 7-OUNCE CAN TUNA PACKED IN OLIVE OIL, UNDRAINED
2 CUPS CANNED CHICKPEAS
¼ CUP CHOPPED FRESH PARSLEY
1 TEASPOON LEMON ZEST
3 TABLESPOONS FRESH LEMON JUICE
1½ TABLESPOONS WHITE WINE VINEGAR
¼ TEASPOON FRESHLY GROUND PEPPER

In a medium mixing bowl, stir together onion, garlic, and oil. Marinate for 1 hour at room temperature. Discard garlic; add tuna and its oil, chickpeas, parsley, lemon zest, lemon juice, vinegar, and pepper. Let marinate for 15 minutes before serving.

Salmon Niçoise Salad

SERVES 4

▶ 487 CALORIES PER SERVING
▶ TOTAL PREPARATION TIME: 30 MINUTES

This take on a classic French bistro dish benefits from the use of high-quality ingredients—from a rich extra-virgin olive oil to farm-fresh lettuce and beans. Typically served with tuna, this recipe calls for salmon, which is a superior source of omega-3 fatty acids. Feel free to swap out chives for parsley or dill, or use a blend of all three.

1 POUND NEW POTATOES
⅓ CUP PLUS 2 TEASPOONS OLIVE OIL
TWO 6-OUNCE SKINLESS SALMON FILLETS
SALT AND FRESHLY GROUND PEPPER
¼ POUND GREEN BEANS
¼ CUP CHOPPED CHIVES
1 TABLESPOON DIJON MUSTARD
1 TABLESPOON FRESH LEMON JUICE
1 HEAD OF BOSTON LETTUCE, LEAVES TORN
2 HARD-BOILED EGGS, HALVED
¼ CUP (ABOUT 2 OUNCES) NIÇOISE OLIVES

1. Preheat broiler.

2. Fill a large saucepan with water; add potatoes. Bring to a boil. Cover, reduce heat, and simmer for 15 minutes, until potatoes are tender. Drain and transfer to a bowl.

3. As the potatoes cook, drizzle 2 teaspoons oil over both sides of the salmon; season with salt and pepper. In a broiler-proof baking dish, broil salmon for 10 to 12 minutes, until cooked through. Remove from heat and set aside.

continued ▶

4. Using the same saucepan as the potatoes, fill with water and add green beans. Bring to a boil and cook for 3 minutes, until beans are tender. Drain, run under cold water, and transfer to a bowl.

5. In a medium mixing bowl, whisk together chives, mustard, lemon juice, and remaining ⅓ cup oil; season with salt. Set aside.

6. After potatoes have cooled, cut them in half. Assemble the salad by starting with a layer of lettuce. Top with potatoes, green beans, salmon, eggs, and olives. Finish with a drizzle of lemon dressing.

Spiced Shrimp Salad with Corn and Black Beans

SERVES 4

▶ 354 CALORIES PER SERVING
▶ TOTAL PREPARATION TIME: 15 MINUTES

If you have a craving for Mexican food, this salad will give you a taste of what you're missing without the fat and calorie traps. Chili powder and ground cumin spice up this shrimp dish, while fresh lemon juice gives it a lively zest.

COOKING SPRAY
1 TABLESPOON CHILI POWDER
½ TEASPOON GARLIC SALT
½ TEASPOON GROUND CUMIN
1½ POUNDS MEDIUM SHRIMP, PEELED AND DEVEINED
2 TABLESPOONS FRESH LIME JUICE
1½ CUPS FROZEN WHOLE-KERNEL CORN, THAWED
¾ CUP JARRED SALSA
¼ CUP CHOPPED FRESH CILANTRO
ONE 15-OUNCE CAN BLACK BEANS, RINSED AND DRAINED

1. Coat a large nonstick skillet with cooking spray; heat over medium-high heat.

2. In a large mixing bowl, whisk together chili powder, garlic salt, and cumin. Add shrimp; toss until evenly coated. Place shrimp in pan; sauté for 3 minutes, until cooked through and pink. Add 1 tablespoon of lime juice to the pan and stir. Transfer shrimp to a plate. Add corn to pan; sauté for 1 minute. Mix in salsa, cilantro, and beans with corn and cook for 1 minute, until heated through. Spoon in remaining 1 tablespoon lime juice. Divide beans among 4 plates; top with shrimp.

Quinoa Salad with Chicken, Walnuts, and Fruit

SERVES 4

▶ 390 CALORIES PER SERVING
▶ TOTAL PREPARATION TIME: 40 MINUTES

Quinoa is a high-fiber, high-protein grain that can be bland when it stands alone, but it marries well with other flavors to make delicious dishes. This recipe also includes walnuts, which are an excellent source of protein, fiber, vitamin E, and omega-3 fatty acids.

COOKING SPRAY
FOUR 4-OUNCE BONELESS, SKINLESS CHICKEN BREASTS
¼ TEASPOON SALT
½ TEASPOON FRESHLY GROUND PEPPER
1½ CUPS WATER
¾ CUP QUINOA
1 TABLESPOON OLIVE OIL
3 TABLESPOONS RED WINE VINEGAR
1 TEASPOON DIJON MUSTARD
1 TABLESPOON FRESH ORANGE JUICE
1 TEASPOON ORANGE ZEST
¼ CUP CHOPPED FRESH MINT
2 GREEN ONIONS, CHOPPED
1 CUP DICED APPLE
½ CUP DRIED CHERRIES
2 TABLESPOONS CHOPPED WALNUTS
½ CUP DICED RED ONION

1. Coat a grill pan or large nonstick skillet with cooking spray and heat over medium-high heat. Season chicken with salt and pepper; cook for 9 minutes, turning once, until no longer pink. Remove from heat and let rest for 2 minutes. Slice into thin strips.

2. While the chicken cooks, pour the water into a medium saucepan and stir in quinoa. Bring water to a boil; reduce heat to medium low, cover, and simmer for 15 minutes. Fluff with a fork and refrigerate for 30 minutes.

3. In a medium mixing bowl, whisk together oil, vinegar, mustard, orange juice, orange zest, mint, and green onions. Stir in apple, cherries, walnuts, and red onion. Combine with quinoa. Divide quinoa among four plates; top with chicken.

Greek Chicken Salad

SERVES 4

▶ 343 CALORIES PER SERVING
▶ TOTAL PREPARATION TIME: 25 MINUTES

The beauty of Greek salad is in its simplicity. Of course, the dish can be served year-round, but it's especially indulgent as a summer salad, when its star ingredients—tomatoes and cucumbers—are at their peak. If you would like to spring for the best olives for the dish, seek out pitted kalamata olives.

⅓ CUP RED WINE VINEGAR

2 TABLESPOONS OLIVE OIL

1 TABLESPOON CHOPPED FRESH DILL (OR 1 TEASPOON DRIED)

1 TEASPOON GARLIC POWDER

¼ TEASPOON SALT

¼ TEASPOON FRESHLY GROUND PEPPER

6 CUPS CHOPPED ROMAINE LETTUCE

2½ CUPS CHOPPED ROTISSERIE CHICKEN

2 MEDIUM TOMATOES, CHOPPED

½ CUP FINELY CHOPPED RED ONION

1 MEDIUM CUCUMBER, PEELED, SEEDED, AND CHOPPED

½ CUP SLICED BLACK OLIVES

½ CUP CRUMBLED FETA CHEESE

In a large bowl, whisk together vinegar, oil, dill, garlic powder, salt, and pepper. Combine with lettuce, chicken, tomatoes, onion, cucumber, olives, and feta; toss until well coated. Serve immediately.

Skirt Steak and Arugula Salad

SERVES 4

▶ 253 CALORIES PER SERVING
▶ TOTAL PREPARATION TIME: 25 MINUTES

If you're looking for a little extra oomph in your salads, opt for arugula, a flavorful leafy green that offers a strong peppery bite. Dressed with a zesty mustard vinaigrette, the salad is the perfect complement to the broiled skirt steak.

1 POUND SKIRT STEAK
SALT AND FRESHLY GROUND PEPPER
2 TEASPOONS DIJON MUSTARD
2 TEASPOONS RED WINE VINEGAR
1 TEASPOON FRESH LEMON JUICE
½ CUP OLIVE OIL
2 TABLESPOONS CHOPPED FRESH CILANTRO
5 CUPS ARUGULA, PACKED
½ RED ONION, THINLY SLICED
8 OUNCES GREEN BEANS, HALVED AND CUT LENGTHWISE
1 BUNCH RADISHES, QUARTERED
1 CUP BEAN SPROUTS
2 CUPS PACKAGED BROCCOLI SLAW
3 GREEN ONIONS, THINLY SLICED

1. Preheat broiler.

2. Season both sides of steak with salt and pepper. On a broiler-proof baking sheet, broil steak for about 4 minutes per side, or until it reaches desired doneness. Remove from heat; let rest for 5 minutes before slicing thinly against the grain.

3. In a large mixing bowl, whisk together mustard, vinegar, lemon juice, oil, cilantro, and a pinch of salt and pepper. Mix in arugula, red onion, green beans, radishes, bean sprouts, broccoli slaw, and green onions; toss until well combined. Divide salad among four plates; top with steak.

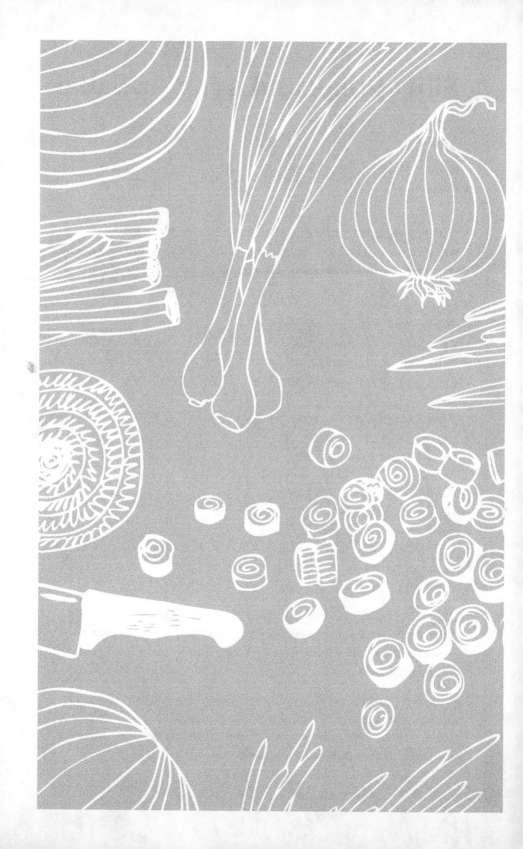

CHAPTER SIX

Snacks

Chai Smoothie

SERVES 1

▶ 246 CALORIES PER SERVING
▶ TOTAL PREPARATION TIME: 40 MINUTES

Chai tea is a mix of black tea, cinnamon, cardamom, black pepper, and other spices. It originated in India, but is now so popular it can be found in most grocery stores.

½ CUP BOILING WATER
¼ CUP SUGAR
4 CHAI TEA BAGS
2 CUPS ICE
½ CUP 1-PERCENT MILK

1. In a small bowl, combine boiling water, sugar, and chai tea bags. Cover and steep 5 minutes. Discard tea bags, then refrigerate tea for 30 minutes or until thoroughly chilled.

2. Place tea, ice, and milk in a blender and process until smooth. Serve immediately.

Citrus Yogurt Parfait

SERVES 4

▶ 180 CALORIES PER SERVING
▶ TOTAL PREPARATION TIME: 5 MINUTES

Greek yogurt is full of protein and makes for a super filling snack. Go with the plain variety and add your own flavors to avoid the extra sugars that come in some yogurts. A good rule of thumb is to choose something sweet, something fruity, and something crunchy. This recipe uses honey, clementines, and pistachios.

3 CUPS PLAIN NONFAT GREEK YOGURT
1 TEASPOON VANILLA EXTRACT
4 TEASPOONS HONEY
28 CLEMENTINE SEGMENTS
¼ CUP SHELLED UNSALTED DRY-ROASTED CHOPPED PISTACHIOS

1. In a medium bowl, combine yogurt and vanilla. Spoon ⅓ cup of yogurt into each of 4 parfait glasses. Top with ½ teaspoon honey, 5 clementine segments, and ½ tablespoon pistachios.

2. Top each parfait with a quarter of remaining yogurt, ½ teaspoon honey, 2 clementine segments, and ½ tablespoon pistachios.

Cinnamon-Sugar Crisps

▶ 89 CALORIES PER SERVING

▶ TOTAL PREPARATION TIME: 20 MINUTES

These chips are surprisingly crunchy and satisfying even though they don't contain oil or butter. Watch them carefully as they bake, since they can easily get burned around the edges.

1 TABLESPOON SUGAR

¼ TEASPOON GROUND CINNAMON

TWO 8-INCH FLOUR TORTILLAS

1 TABLESPOON WATER

1. Preheat oven to 350°F.

2. In a small bowl, combine sugar and cinnamon. Lightly brush both sides of tortillas with water and sprinkle each side with the cinnamon-sugar mixture. Cut each tortilla into 12 wedges and arrange in a single layer on a cookie sheet. Bake 15 minutes or until crisp. Let cookies cool on a wire rack before serving.

Plantain Chips

SERVES 4

▶ 190 CALORIES PER SERVING
▶ TOTAL PREPARATION TIME: 9 MINUTES

Plantains may look like large bananas, but they have to be cooked before you eat them. They can also be a bit tough to peel, so use a sharp knife and be careful. They contain vitamins A and C, along with other nutrients.

1 TABLESPOON OLIVE OIL
2 PLANTAINS, PEELED AND CUT INTO ¼-INCH DIAGONAL SLICES
¼ TEASPOON SALT
⅛ TEASPOON GROUND RED PEPPER

In a large nonstick skillet, heat oil over medium heat. Add plantain slices and cook 3 minutes on each side or until brown and crispy. Remove from pan and sprinkle with salt and pepper before serving.

Glazed Dried Fruit and Nuts

SERVES 4

▶ 388 CALORIES PER SERVING
▶ TOTAL PREPARATION TIME: 15 MINUTES

Think of this as trail mix kicked up a notch. Use whatever kinds of nuts, seeds, and dried fruit you like—it's completely customizable based on your preferences. Buy the nuts pre-chopped to save on prep time.

COOKING SPRAY
1 TEASPOON UNSALTED BUTTER
¼ CUP HONEY
¼ CUP SLIVERED ALMONDS
¼ CUP CHOPPED HAZELNUTS
¼ CUP CHOPPED PECANS
¼ CUP SUNFLOWER SEEDS
½ TEASPOON GROUND CINNAMON
¼ TEASPOON SALT
¼ TEASPOON GROUND CARDAMOM
DASH OF GROUND CLOVES
1 CUP RAISINS

1. Line a baking sheet with parchment paper or foil. Coat it with cooking spray and set aside.

2. In a large nonstick skillet, heat butter over medium-high heat. Stir in honey and cook 2 minutes or until it starts to bubble around the edges. Add almonds, hazelnuts, pecans, sunflower seeds, cinnamon, salt, cardamom, and cloves. Cook over medium heat for 8 minutes or until nuts turn golden, stirring frequently. Add raisins, spread onto baking sheet, and cool completely before serving.

Sweet and Spicy Roasted Nuts

SERVES 4

▶ 180 CALORIES PER SERVING
▶ TOTAL PREPARATION TIME: 23 MINUTES

Roasted nuts are nothing new, but these shine with Indian spices like cardamom and cloves. Nuts are a great snack because they have protein and heart-healthy unsaturated fat, meaning they'll keep you full until your next meal. Like things a little spicier? Add some ground red pepper to the mix.

1½ TEASPOONS PACKED BROWN SUGAR
1½ TEASPOONS HONEY
1 TEASPOON CANOLA OIL
¾ TEASPOON GROUND CINNAMON
⅛ TEASPOON SALT
⅛ TEASPOON GROUND CARDAMOM
⅛ TEASPOON GROUND CLOVES
DASH OF FRESHLY GROUND PEPPER
¼ CUP BLANCHED ALMONDS
¼ CUP CASHEWS
¼ CUP HAZELNUTS

1. Preheat oven to 350°F.

2. In a medium microwave-safe bowl, combine brown sugar, honey, oil, cinnamon, salt, cardamom, cloves, and pepper. Microwave for 30 seconds and stir. Add nuts to sugar mixture and toss to coat.

3. Line a baking sheet with parchment paper and spread nuts evenly. Bake for 15 minutes or until golden brown. Cool before serving.

Peanut Butter Oatmeal Balls

SERVES 4

▶ 260 CALORIES PER SERVING
▶ TOTAL PREPARATION TIME: 25 MINUTES

These are the perfect energizing bites—they have fiber, protein, and healthy fat to keep you satisfied. If you don't like peanuts, roll them in any other crushed nut you'd like. These are tasty at room temperature or cold from the refrigerator.

¼ CUP OLD-FASHIONED ROLLED OATS

1 TABLESPOON CHOPPED ALMONDS

1 TABLESPOON GROUND FLAXSEED

1½ TEASPOONS CHIA SEEDS

PINCH OF CINNAMON

PINCH OF SALT

1½ TABLESPOONS CREAMY PEANUT BUTTER

1 TABLESPOON HONEY

DASH OF VANILLA EXTRACT

1 TABLESPOON MINI CHOCOLATE CHIPS

½ CUP CRUSHED PEANUTS FOR COATING THE BALLS

1. In a large bowl, stir together oats, almonds, flaxseed, chia seeds, cinnamon, and salt.

2. Place the peanut butter in a microwave-safe bowl and microwave for 20 to 30 seconds or until melted; allow to cool slightly. Stir in honey and vanilla, and pour peanut butter mixture over oats. Once mixture is combined and sticking together, fold in chocolate chips.

3. Using your hands, roll dough into four balls, then roll them in the crushed peanuts.

Peanut Butter and Banana Roll-Ups

SERVES 4

▶ 367 CALORIES PER SERVING
▶ TOTAL PREPARATION TIME: 8 MINUTES

The winning combination of peanut butter and bananas is rolled up in a whole-wheat tortilla, making a perfectly portable snack. The wheat germ can be omitted if you don't have it, but it adds crunch, protein, and fiber.

½ CUP REDUCED-FAT PEANUT BUTTER
⅓ CUP VANILLA LOW-FAT YOGURT
2 BANANAS, SLICED
1 TABLESPOON ORANGE JUICE
FOUR 8-INCH FAT-FREE WHOLE-WHEAT TORTILLAS
2 TABLESPOONS HONEY-CRUNCH WHEAT GERM
¼ TEASPOON GROUND CINNAMON

1. In a small bowl, combine peanut butter and yogurt and stir until smooth. In another small bowl, toss bananas with orange juice.

2. Spread about 3 tablespoons of the peanut butter mixture over each tortilla, leaving ½ inch bare around the edges. Arrange about ⅓ cup banana slices in a single layer on top.

3. In a small bowl, combine wheat germ and cinnamon. Sprinkle over banana slices, roll up, and slice each into 6 pieces.

Open-Faced Pear, Peanut Butter, and Cream Cheese Sandwiches

SERVES 4

▶ 355 CALORIES PER SERVING
▶ TOTAL PREPARATION TIME: 12 MINUTES

A perfect snack has some carbohydrates, fat, and protein. This one hits all those points and more. If you can't find an Anjou pear, opt for an Asian pear or apple.

¼ CUP CREAM CHEESE, SOFTENED
1 TABLESPOON MAPLE SYRUP
¼ TEASPOON GROUND CINNAMON
PINCH OF SALT
4 SLICES CINNAMON-RAISIN BREAD, TOASTED
½ CUP CRUNCHY PEANUT BUTTER
1 ANJOU PEAR, THINLY SLICED

1. In a medium bowl, stir together cream cheese, maple syrup, cinnamon, and salt.

2. On each slice of bread, spread 2 tablespoons peanut butter and 1 tablespoon cream cheese mixture. Top with pear slices.

Blue Cheese–Stuffed Figs with Prosciutto

SERVES 4

▶ 263 CALORIES PER SERVING
▶ TOTAL PREPARATION TIME: 12 MINUTES

While these could be served uncooked, the flavors are heightened when the figs are exposed to heat. Make sure the grill is at a medium-high heat—you want to crisp up the prosciutto and lightly melt the blue cheese.

½ CUP BLUE CHEESE, CUT INTO 16 CUBES
8 BLACK MISSION FIGS, HALVED
8 SLICES PROSCIUTTO, HALVED LENGTHWISE
2 TABLESPOONS OLIVE OIL
SALT AND FRESHLY GROUND PEPPER

1. Preheat grill to medium-high heat. Place a piece of blue cheese on each fig half. Wrap a piece of prosciutto around each fig half, overlapping the ends and making sure to cover the cheese.

2. Grill figs until prosciutto begins to crisp up, about 2 minutes on each side. Lightly drizzle warm figs with oil and season with salt and pepper before serving.

Cheesy Garlic Popcorn

SERVES 3

▶ 250 CALORIES PER SERVING
▶ TOTAL PREPARATION TIME: 5 MINUTES

Popcorn is a healthy snack that can carry all sorts of different flavors. To make plain popcorn without an air popper, place kernels in a glass bowl and microwave for 4 to 5 minutes or until the popping slows.

1 TABLESPOON UNSALTED BUTTER
1 TABLESPOON OLIVE OIL
1 GARLIC CLOVE, PRESSED
½ TEASPOON DRIED THYME
¼ TEASPOON DRIED BASIL
8 CUPS PLAIN POPPED POPCORN
¾ CUP GRATED PARMESAN CHEESE

1. In a small saucepan, melt butter with the oil and garlic over medium-low heat. Cook, stirring frequently, for 1 to 2 minutes or until garlic is soft. Add thyme and basil and stir.

2. Put popcorn in a large bowl and drizzle with butter mixture while stirring with a large spoon. Once popcorn is evenly coated, add cheese and toss well.

Crunchy Mozzarella Nuggets

SERVES 4

▶ 91 CALORIES PER SERVING

▶ TOTAL PREPARATION TIME: 10 MINUTES

Everybody loves mozzarella sticks, but the deep-fried appetizer isn't part of a healthful diet. This version uses prepackaged string cheese and calls for baking over frying.

⅓ CUP PANKO BREAD CRUMBS

3 TABLESPOONS EGG SUBSTITUTE

THREE 1-OUNCE PART-SKIM MOZZARELLA STRING-CHEESE STICKS

COOKING SPRAY

¼ CUP LOWER-SODIUM MARINARA SAUCE FOR DIPPING

1. Preheat oven to 425°F.

2. In a medium skillet over medium heat, toast the bread crumbs for 2 minutes, stirring frequently. Place bread crumbs in a shallow dish. Pour egg substitute into another shallow dish.

3. Cut mozzarella sticks into 1-inch pieces. Working with one piece at a time, dip cheese in egg substitute and then in bread crumbs.

4. Coat a baking sheet with cooking spray and place cheese on it. Bake for 3 minutes or until cheese is softened and warmed through.

5. Microwave marinara sauce for 1 minute, stirring halfway through. Serve mozzarella pieces with the dipping sauce.

Jalapeño Poppers

SERVES 4

▶ 255 CALORIES PER SERVING
▶ TOTAL PREPARATION TIME: 15 MINUTES

Another great appetizer or snack, jalapeño poppers can be a bit high in fat and calories when deep fried. These are baked to lighten the load. When you're seeding the jalapeños, make sure to get rid of the ribs as well, since those can carry heat, too.

4 OUNCES CREAM CHEESE, SOFTENED
½ CUP GRATED SHARP CHEDDAR CHEESE
SALT AND FRESHLY GROUND PEPPER
6 JALAPEÑOS, HALVED, SEEDED, AND DERIBBED

1. Preheat oven to 450°F.

2. In a small bowl, mix together cream cheese and cheddar. Season with salt and pepper. Take each jalapeño half and fill with about 1 tablespoon of cheese mixture.

3. Line a baking sheet with parchment paper and place the stuffed peppers on it. Bake for 10 minutes or until cheese is browned and bubbly, rotating sheet halfway through. Let cool slightly before serving.

Nachos with Everything

SERVES 4

▶ 412 CALORIES PER SERVING

▶ TOTAL PREPARATION TIME: 30 MINUTES

By loading up each chip with toppings instead of just piling the ingredients onto one another, you guarantee that every bite will have all the flavors represented. Using baked tortilla chips cuts down on the fat, and with all the toppings, you'll never notice.

8 OUNCES LEAN GROUND BEEF

½ CUP CHOPPED JARRED ROASTED RED BELL PEPPERS

1 TEASPOON CHILI POWDER

½ TEASPOON DRIED OREGANO

¼ TEASPOON SALT

ONE 14.5-OUNCE CAN NO-SALT-ADDED DICED TOMATOES, UNDRAINED

1 GARLIC CLOVE, CRUSHED

COOKING SPRAY

ONE 16-OUNCE CAN FAT-FREE REFRIED BEANS WITH MILD CHILES

¼ CUP MINCED FRESH CILANTRO, DIVIDED

¼ CUP CHOPPED GREEN ONIONS, DIVIDED

26 BAKED TORTILLA CHIPS

1 CUP SHREDDED MONTEREY JACK CHEESE

3 TABLESPOONS LOW-FAT SOUR CREAM

1. Preheat oven to 375°F.

2. In a large nonstick skillet, cook meat over medium-high heat until browned, stirring to break it up, about 10 minutes. Add bell peppers, chili powder, oregano, salt, tomatoes, and garlic. Cook for 8 minutes or until thick, stirring occasionally.

continued ▶

3.Place another skillet coated with cooking spray over medium heat until hot. Add beans, 2 tablespoons cilantro, and 2 tablespoons green onions. Cook 2 minutes or until heated through. Place chips on a baking sheet in a single layer. Spread warm bean mixture over each chip and top with meat and cheese. Bake for 9 minutes or until cheese melts.

4. Top with sour cream, remaining cilantro, and remaining green onions; serve immediately.

Boneless Chicken Wings

SERVES 4

▶ 493 CALORIES PER SERVING
▶ TOTAL PREPARATION TIME: 40 MINUTES

Pan-frying the chicken tenders gives them a nice crispy texture, but without all the oil that comes from deep-frying them. And instead of buffalo sauce, which is almost all butter, this vinegar-based version is much lighter. Don't know which hot sauce to use? Frank's RedHot is a good choice.

⅔ CUP REDUCED-FAT SOUR CREAM

½ CUP CRUMBLED BLUE CHEESE

4 TABLESPOONS WHITE VINEGAR

¾ TEASPOON CAYENNE PEPPER, DIVIDED

3 TABLESPOONS NONFAT BUTTERMILK

3 TABLESPOONS HOT SAUCE

2 POUNDS CHICKEN TENDERS

6 TABLESPOONS WHOLE-WHEAT FLOUR

6 TABLESPOONS CORNMEAL

2 TABLESPOONS CANOLA OIL

2 CUPS CARROT STICKS

2 CUPS CELERY STICKS

1. In a small bowl, whisk together sour cream, blue cheese, 1 tablespoon vinegar, and ¼ teaspoon cayenne pepper. Cover and refrigerate.

2. In a large bowl, whisk together buttermilk, 2 tablespoons hot sauce, and 2 tablespoons vinegar. Add chicken and toss to coat. Refrigerate for 10 minutes to let flavors sink in.

3. In a shallow dish, whisk together flour and cornmeal.

continued ▶

4. In a small bowl, whisk together remaining 1 tablespoon hot sauce and remaining 1 tablespoon vinegar.

5. Remove chicken from marinade and roll in flour mixture until evenly coated. Sprinkle both sides of chicken with remaining ½ teaspoon cayenne.

6. In a large nonstick skillet over medium heat, heat 1 tablespoon oil. Add half the chicken pieces and cook until golden brown and cooked through, 3 to 4 minutes per side. Repeat with remaining 1 tablespoon of oil and chicken. Drizzle chicken with reserved hot sauce mixture and serve with sour cream dip, carrots, and celery.

CHAPTER SEVEN

Lunch and Dinner

Parmesan-Crusted Portobello Caps

SERVES 4

▶ 94 CALORIES PER SERVING
▶ TOTAL PREPARATION TIME: 20 MINUTES

Sharp, hard cheese is a dieter's friend. Adding even a dash to dishes gives a boost of flavor without adding too many calories. This recipe combines savory Parmesan with meaty mushrooms, making it a satisfying low-cal meal.

2 TABLESPOONS FRESHLY GRATED PARMESAN CHEESE
1 TABLESPOON MINCED FRESH BASIL (OR 1 TEASPOON DRIED)
1 EGG, LIGHTLY BEATEN
1 EGG WHITE, LIGHTLY BEATEN
4 PORTOBELLO MUSHROOM CAPS
2 TABLESPOONS ALL-PURPOSE FLOUR
1 TABLESPOON OLIVE OIL
2 TABLESPOONS FRESH LEMON JUICE

1. Preheat oven to 400°F.

2. In a small mixing bowl, combine Parmesan, basil, egg, and egg white.

3. In a sealable plastic bag, gently shake mushrooms with flour until they are coated.

4. In a large nonstick skillet, heat oil over medium heat. Dip mushrooms in egg mixture. Sauté mushrooms in skillet for 2 minutes on each side, until light brown. Sprinkle lemon juice over mushrooms. Remove from pan.

5. Place mushrooms in a baking dish and bake for 10 minutes or until tender. Let cool slightly before serving.

Grilled Cheese and Tomato Sandwich

▶ 300 CALORIES PER SERVING
▶ TOTAL PREPARATION TIME: 10 MINUTES

Inspired by the classic duo of grilled cheese and tomato soup, this sandwich will satisfy your cravings for comfort food. Rather than prepping the sandwich for pan-frying with butter, this recipe calls for heart-healthy canola oil, which is low in saturated fat.

2 SLICES WHOLE-WHEAT BREAD
1 TABLESPOON CANOLA OIL
1 SLICE (ABOUT 1 OUNCE) REDUCED-FAT PROVOLONE CHEESE
1 TEASPOON WHOLE-GRAIN MUSTARD
¼ CUP BABY SPINACH
1 TOMATO, THINLY SLICED

1. Using a pastry brush, coat one side of each piece of bread with oil. With oiled side facing down, top one slice with cheese, mustard, spinach, and tomato. Top with remaining slice of bread, oiled side facing up.

2. Heat a cast-iron or heavy skillet over medium heat for about 3 minutes. Using a spatula, transfer sandwich to the pan. Cook for 1 minute while pressing sandwich into skillet with the spatula, until bottom is browned. Flip over sandwich and repeat step; cheese should be melted. Cut sandwich in half and serve.

Black Bean and Cheese Quesadillas

SERVES 4

▶ 377 CALORIES PER SERVING
▶ TOTAL PREPARATION TIME: 15 MINUTES

If your new healthy lifestyle is causing you to miss out on taco night, then throw your own kind of fiesta with these fiber- and protein-rich quesadillas. The best part about this dish is that you can prep dinner for four in a flash, giving a new meaning to fast food.

ONE 15-OUNCE CAN BLACK BEANS, DRAINED AND RINSED
½ CUP SHREDDED MONTEREY JACK CHEESE
½ CUP PREPARED FRESH SALSA
FOUR 8-INCH WHOLE-WHEAT TORTILLAS
2 TEASPOONS CANOLA OIL
1 AVOCADO, DICED

1. In a medium bowl, stir together beans, cheese, and ¼ cup salsa. Lay out each tortilla; spread ½ cup of bean mixture on half of each tortilla. Fold over tortillas, pressing together gently.

2. In a large nonstick skillet, heat 1 teaspoon oil over medium heat. Cook two quesadillas at a time, 2 minutes per side, until golden brown. Remove from heat. Repeat steps with remaining quesadillas.

3. To serve, top quesadillas with remaining ¼ cup salsa and avocado.

Roasted Veggie and Bean Tostadas with Cheese

SERVES 4

▶ 463 CALORIES PER SERVING

▶ TOTAL PREPARATION TIME: 50 MINUTES

Roasting your vegetables is a great way to get maximum flavor from them while dedicating minimal time to cooking them. Any leftover veggies from this dish will work well the next day when stirred into a scramble or folded into an omelet.

10 OUNCES BUTTON MUSHROOMS, TRIMMED AND QUARTERED

2 ZUCCHINI, THINLY SLICED LENGTHWISE

2 RED BELL PEPPERS, SEEDED AND CHOPPED INTO 1½-INCH PIECES

3 TABLESPOONS OLIVE OIL

SALT

8 SMALL CORN TORTILLAS

ONE 15-OUNCE CAN REFRIED BEANS

4 OUNCES (ABOUT 1 CUP) GRATED CHEDDAR CHEESE

4 TABLESPOONS LOW-FAT SOUR CREAM (OPTIONAL)

FRESH CILANTRO LEAVES (OPTIONAL)

HOT SAUCE (OPTIONAL)

1. Preheat oven to 450°F.

2. Divide mushrooms, zucchini, and bell peppers between two baking sheets. Toss each batch with 1 tablespoon oil and season with salt. Roast vegetables for 20 to 25 minutes, until tender, stirring each batch midway through roasting and swapping the placement of the baking sheets. Remove vegetables from oven; set aside in a medium bowl.

3. Using the same baking sheets, arrange the tortillas and brush one side of each tortilla with the remaining tablespoon of oil. Divide the refried beans and cheese among the tortillas. Bake for 5 to 7 minutes, until beans are warm and cheese has melted. Spoon out the vegetables onto each tortilla; top each with a dollop of sour cream, a pinch of cilantro, and a splash of hot sauce, if using.

Butternut Squash Barley Risotto

SERVES 4

▶ 427 CALORIES PER SERVING

▶ TOTAL PREPARATION TIME: 50 MINUTES

When limiting calories in your diet, it's a smart choice to eat more whole grains, since they suppress your appetite by keeping you feeling full for a longer period of time. Replacing regular risotto in this recipe, barley lowers blood cholesterol levels, helps maintain blood sugar levels, and eases digestion.

2 TABLESPOONS OLIVE OIL

1 BUTTERNUT SQUASH (ABOUT 1½ POUNDS), PEELED, SEEDED, AND
    CHOPPED INTO 1-INCH PIECES

1 ONION, FINELY CHOPPED

¾ TEASPOON SALT, DIVIDED

¼ TEASPOON FRESHLY GROUND PEPPER, DIVIDED

1 CUP PEARL BARLEY

½ CUP DRY WHITE WINE

3 CUPS LOW-SODIUM VEGETABLE BROTH

1 CUP PACKED BABY SPINACH

½ CUP (ABOUT 2 OUNCES) GRATED FRESH PARMESAN CHEESE

1 TABLESPOON UNSALTED BUTTER

1. Preheat oven to 400°F.

2. In a Dutch oven or heavy oven-safe pot, heat oil over medium heat. Sauté squash, onion, salt, and pepper for 5 minutes, until onion softens, stirring often. Mix in barley and cook for 1 minute. Pour in wine; cook for 1 minute, stirring constantly, until liquid evaporates. Pour in broth and bring to a boil; cover and place pot in oven. Bake for 35 to 40 minutes, until barley is tender.

3. Remove from oven. Stir in spinach, Parmesan, and butter; serve immediately.

Eggplant and Ricotta Lasagna

SERVES 4

▶ 378 CALORIES PER SERVING
▶ TOTAL PREPARATION TIME: 30 MINUTES

Eggplant Parmesan may be a thing of the past for you, but this cheesy baked dish may help you battle a craving for it. This no-noodle recipe is also a great pick for carb-conscious dieters and reluctant veggie eaters.

½ POUND PLUM TOMATOES, HALVED AND SEEDED
1 GARLIC CLOVE
4 TABLESPOONS OLIVE OIL
1 TEASPOON SALT, DIVIDED
¾ TEASPOON FRESHLY GROUND PEPPER, DIVIDED
2 EGGPLANTS (ABOUT 1½ POUNDS EACH), CUT LENGTHWISE INTO
    ¼-INCH SLICES
1 CUP RICOTTA
1 EGG
½ CUP CHOPPED FRESH BASIL
¼ CUP FRESHLY GRATED PARMESAN OR ASIAGO CHEESE
4 CUPS MIXED GREENS

1. Preheat broiler.

2. In a food processor or blender, pulse together tomatoes, garlic, 1 tablespoon oil, ¼ teaspoon salt, and ¼ teaspoon pepper.

3. Divide 2 tablespoons of oil among the eggplant slices; evenly coat them using a pastry brush. Season each side with ½ teaspoon salt and ¼ teaspoon pepper. On a broiler-proof baking sheet, place eggplant slices in a single layer and broil 3 to 4 minutes on each side, until tender and charred.

4. Set oven to 400°F.

continued ▶

5. In a small mixing bowl, stir together ricotta, egg, basil, remaining ¼ teaspoon salt, and remaining ¼ teaspoon pepper, until well combined.

6. Using an 8-inch square baking dish, pour in half of the tomato sauce and spread evenly. Create a single layer of eggplant using one-third of the slices. Spread half the ricotta mixture on top of the eggplant layer. Top with a single layer of eggplant, using one-third of the slices. Spread the remaining ricotta on top of this layer. Finish with a final layer of eggplant. Spread Parmesan evenly across the top layer.

7. Bake the lasagna for 15 to 20 minutes, until bubbling. Remove from heat and let stand for 10 minutes before serving.

8. Divide mixed greens among plates. Sprinkle each serving with remaining 1 tablespoon oil; season with salt and pepper. Serve alongside lasagna.

Whole-Wheat Spaghetti Carbonara

SERVES 4

▶ 385 CALORIES PER SERVING
▶ TOTAL PREPARATION TIME: 30 MINUTES

You may be watching what you eat, but you're allowed to enjoy the good stuff in moderation. Bacon makes an appearance in this dish, which proves that a little goes a long way in terms of flavor. If you only have regular pasta on hand, feel free to use it, but know that going for the whole-wheat variety accounts for almost 10 grams of fiber per serving.

8 OUNCES WHOLE-WHEAT SPAGHETTI
2 CUPS FROZEN PEAS, THAWED
3 GARLIC CLOVES, MINCED
4 STRIPS THICK-CUT BACON
2 EGGS, ROOM TEMPERATURE
¾ CUP FINELY SHREDDED PARMESAN CHEESE, DIVIDED
¼ TEASPOON SALT
¼ TEASPOON FRESHLY GROUND PEPPER

1. In a large saucepan, bring water to a boil. Drop in spaghetti; cook for about 8 minutes until pasta is tender (refer to package directions for accurate cooking time). After cooking for 5 minutes, stir in peas and garlic.

2. As the pasta cooks, use a nonstick skillet to cook bacon over medium heat. Transfer bacon to a plate lined with paper towels to soak up the grease. In a large bowl, whisk together reserved bacon drippings, eggs, ½ cup Parmesan, salt, and pepper. Chop bacon and stir into egg mixture.

3. When the pasta and peas are done, strain and reserve ¾ cup of cooking water. Stir pasta, peas, and water into egg mixture, quickly, until well combined. Let stand 5 minutes, until sauce has thickened; stir occasionally. Divide the pasta among 4 bowls and sprinkle the remaining ¼ cup Parmesan over top before serving.

Lemon-Garlic Shrimp

SERVES 4

▶ 117 CALORIES PER SERVING
▶ TOTAL PREPARATION TIME: 16 MINUTES

The fragrant blend of lemon and garlic can do no wrong when it comes to flavoring a meal. Throw butter into the mix, as this recipe does, and you have yourself a winning dish. If you can't find lemon-pepper seasoning, you can finish the shrimp with a squeeze of fresh lemon.

COOKING SPRAY
1¼ POUNDS LARGE SHRIMP, PEELED AND DEVEINED
¼ CUP FRESH LEMON JUICE
2 TABLESPOONS UNSALTED BUTTER, MELTED
3 GARLIC CLOVES, MINCED
1 TEASPOON WORCESTERSHIRE SAUCE
¾ TEASPOON LEMON-PEPPER SEASONING
¼ TEASPOON GROUND RED PEPPER
2 TABLESPOONS CHOPPED FRESH PARSLEY

1. Preheat oven to 425°F.

2. Coat a 9-by-13-inch baking dish with cooking spray. Place shrimp in dish in a single layer.

3. In a small mixing bowl, whisk together lemon juice, butter, garlic, Worcestershire sauce, lemon-pepper seasoning, and red pepper. Pour mixture over shrimp.

4. Bake shrimp for 9 minutes, or until shrimp are pink and cooked through. Remove from heat; sprinkle parsley over shrimp, and serve.

Shrimp and Jalapeño Ceviche

SERVES 4

▶ 80 CALORIES PER SERVING
▶ TOTAL PREPARATION TIME: 35 MINUTES

Tantalizing the palate with a combination of citrus and spice, this chilled dish is a harmonious blend of big flavors and very few calories. If you have trouble finding jicama, feel free to substitute with julienned radishes, but know that the latter are more peppery.

½ POUND PEELED LARGE SHRIMP, COOKED

2 TABLESPOONS FRESH LIME JUICE

2 TABLESPOONS CHOPPED FRESH CILANTRO

½ GARLIC CLOVE, MINCED

1 GREEN ONION, CHOPPED

½ RED BELL PEPPER, SEEDED, DERIBBED, AND DICED

½ CUP PEELED CHOPPED JICAMA

¼ CUP ORANGE SECTIONS

½ JALAPEÑO, SEEDED, DERIBBED, AND MINCED

PINCH OF SALT

In a large mixing bowl, combine all ingredients. Chill for at least 30 minutes. Serve cold.

Spicy Baked Tilapia

SERVES 4

▶ 230 CALORIES PER SERVING
▶ TOTAL PREPARATION TIME: 14 MINUTES

Healthy cooking doesn't need to be bland. Dip into your spice rack to amp up your dishes while keeping calorie counts low. The chili spice blend in this recipe sasses up typically mild, delicate tilapia for a more exciting meal.

1 TEASPOON CHILI POWDER
¼ TEASPOON CAYENNE PEPPER
1 TEASPOON GARLIC POWDER
1 TEASPOON SALT
½ TEASPOON FRESHLY GROUND PEPPER
FOUR 6-OUNCE TILAPIA FILLETS
2 TABLESPOONS OLIVE OIL
LIME WEDGES (OPTIONAL)

1. Preheat oven to 450°F.

2. In a small mixing bowl, combine chili powder, cayenne pepper, garlic powder, salt, and pepper. Divide spice mix evenly over both sides of tilapia fillets.

3. Coat a baking sheet with 1 tablespoon oil. Place fish on the baking sheet in a single layer. Drizzle remaining 1 tablespoon oil over the fish. Bake for 8 minutes, or until fish is golden brown and flaking. Serve with lime wedges (if using).

Lemon-Caper Spaghetti with Salmon

SERVES 4

▶ 462 CALORIES PER SERVING

▶ TOTAL PREPARATION TIME: 20 MINUTES

From the whole-grain pasta to the lean protein to the side of spinach, this recipe helps you bring together a close-to-perfect meal in only 20 minutes. The dish calls for lemon zest to be mixed into the pasta, which is worth adding for the bright boost of concentrated citrus flavor it gives the plate.

½ POUND WHOLE-WHEAT SPAGHETTI

1 GARLIC CLOVE, MINCED

3 TABLESPOONS OLIVE OIL

½ TEASPOON SALT

½ TEASPOON FRESHLY GROUND PEPPER

¼ CUP CHOPPED FRESH BASIL LEAVES

3 TABLESPOONS CAPERS

ZEST OF 1 LEMON

2 TABLESPOONS FRESH LEMON JUICE

FOUR 4-OUNCE SALMON FILLETS

2 CUPS PACKED BABY SPINACH

1. In a large stockpot or saucepan, bring salted water to a boil over high heat. Add the spaghetti and cook for about 8 minutes until pasta is al dente (refer to package directions for accurate cooking time). Drain pasta and pour into a large mixing bowl. Add garlic, 2 tablespoons oil, salt, and pepper; mix until well combined. Stir in basil, capers, lemon zest, and lemon juice; mix until well combined.

continued ▶

2. In a large nonstick skillet, heat remaining tablespoon of oil over medium-high heat. Season the salmon with salt and pepper; cook for 2 minutes on each side, until medium rare. Transfer salmon to dish.

3. Arrange servings by placing ½ cup of spinach in each bowl. Top with one-quarter of the spaghetti mixture, and finish with a piece of salmon.

Honey-Soy Broiled Salmon with Spinach and Pepper Sauté

SERVES 4

▶ 321 CALORIES PER SERVING

▶ TOTAL PREPARATION TIME: 20 MINUTES

This dish is a great choice if you want to cook a meal that will impress your family and friends but you just don't have the time to slave over the stove. A real crowd pleaser, the honey and soy glaze will give the fish a sweet and savory crust while it adds some excitement to your side of wilted greens.

1 TABLESPOON HONEY

3 TEASPOONS LOW-SODIUM SOY SAUCE

1¼-POUND PIECE OF SKINLESS SALMON FILLET, CUT INTO 4 PIECES

SALT AND FRESHLY GROUND PEPPER

1 TABLESPOON CANOLA OIL

1 RED BELL PEPPER, SEEDED AND THINLY SLICED

1 TABLESPOON CHOPPED FRESH GINGER

12 CUPS PACKED SPINACH

1. Preheat broiler. In a small mixing bowl, whisk together honey and 1 teaspoon soy sauce. Set aside.

2. Line a broiler-proof baking dish with aluminum foil. Season salmon with salt and pepper. Place salmon on dish and broil for 5 minutes. Pour honey mixture over salmon and broil for another 2 to 5 minutes, until cooked through and flaky.

3. While salmon broils, use a large nonstick skillet to heat oil over medium-high heat. Sauté bell pepper for 3 to 4 minutes, until softened. Stir in ginger until well combined. Add spinach and season with salt; sauté for 2 minutes, until wilted. Stir in the remaining 2 teaspoons soy sauce. Serve alongside salmon.

Smoked Salmon and Cream Cheese Wraps with Spinach and Artichokes

SERVES 4

▶ 397 CALORIES PER SERVING
▶ TOTAL PREPARATION TIME: 12 MINUTES

With fiber-rich whole-wheat wraps, omega-3-filled smoked salmon, and vitamin-packed spinach, this dish is a heart-healthy power recipe. Boasting 43 grams of protein per serving, these wraps will also keep you feeling full.

½ CUP REDUCED-FAT CREAM CHEESE

2 TABLESPOONS CHOPPED FRESH DILL

2 TABLESPOONS CHOPPED FRESH CHIVES

¼ TEASPOON FRESHLY GROUND PEPPER

4 WHOLE-GRAIN WRAPS

8 OUNCES SMOKED SALMON

2 TABLESPOONS CAPERS

3 TABLESPOONS SUNFLOWER SEEDS

1 CUP SLICED ARTICHOKE HEARTS

2 CUPS PACKED BABY SPINACH

In a large mixing bowl, combine cream cheese, dill, chives, and pepper. Divide mixture among wraps and spread evenly. To finish assembling sandwiches, layer one-fourth of the salmon, capers, sunflower seeds, artichoke hearts, and spinach in each wrap. Roll wraps tightly; cut each in half.

Pan-Fried Chicken Breasts

SERVES 4

▶ 92 CALORIES PER SERVING
▶ TOTAL PREPARATION TIME: 13 MINUTES

Simple and versatile, these chicken breasts can be prepped in bulk and kept in the refrigerator to be used throughout the week in everything from omelets to salads. For a flavorful, low-calorie accompaniment to this dish, lightly dress a bed of arugula with salt, pepper, and a squeeze of lemon. The recipe calls for you to pound out the chicken breasts, which will allow them to cook more quickly and evenly.

FOUR 4-OUNCE BONELESS, SKINLESS CHICKEN BREASTS, HALVED
½ TEASPOON SALT
½ TEASPOON FRESHLY GROUND PEPPER
2 TEASPOONS OLIVE OIL

1. Place chicken breasts between two pieces of heavy-duty plastic wrap. Using a meat mallet or rolling pin, pound out the chicken breasts until they are about ½ inch thick. Season both sides with salt and pepper.

2. In a large nonstick skillet, heat oil over medium-high heat. Sauté chicken for about 3 minutes on each side, until light brown and cooked through.

Breaded Chicken Thighs with Lemon and Garlic

SERVES 4

▶ 172 CALORIES PER SERVING

▶ TOTAL PREPARATION TIME: 26 MINUTES

Chicken breasts may be the leanest cut of the bird, but that doesn't mean they're the only part you can use when making healthy dishes. If you want more taste out of your chicken dish, go to the dark side. Thighs are a bit higher in calories, but are juicier, more tender, and even cheaper than chicken breasts.

4 CHICKEN THIGHS, SKINNED

1 TABLESPOON ALL-PURPOSE FLOUR

¼ TEASPOON SALT

¼ TEASPOON FRESHLY GROUND PEPPER

1 EGG WHITE, LIGHTLY BEATEN

1 TEASPOON WATER

½ CUP ITALIAN-SEASONED BREAD CRUMBS

2 TEASPOONS OLIVE OIL

½ CUP FAT-FREE, LOW-SODIUM CHICKEN BROTH

½ CUP WHITE WINE

2 TABLESPOONS FRESH LEMON JUICE

2 GARLIC CLOVES, FINELY MINCED

2 TABLESPOONS CHOPPED FRESH PARSLEY

1 TABLESPOON CAPERS, DRAINED

1. In a heavy-duty sealable plastic bag, combine chicken with flour, salt, and pepper. Shake bag to coat chicken evenly. In a shallow bowl, whisk together egg white and water. In a separate shallow bowl, place bread crumbs.

2. Remove 1 chicken thigh from bag, dip in egg white mixture, then dredge in bread crumbs. Set aside. Repeat steps with remaining chicken.

3. In a large nonstick skillet, heat oil over medium heat. Starting with the bone side up, cook chicken 3 minutes on each side, or until browned. Add broth, wine, lemon juice, and garlic to pan with chicken, and bring to a boil. Reduce heat and cover; simmer for 8 minutes. Add parsley and capers to pan; simmer uncovered for 5 minutes, until chicken is cooked through. Serve immediately.

Goat Cheese–Stuffed Chicken Breasts with Sun-Dried Tomatoes

SERVES 4

▶ 296 CALORIES PER SERVING
▶ TOTAL PREPARATION TIME: 55 MINUTES

Just because you're being mindful of calories doesn't mean that you need to eliminate cheese from your diet. Goat cheese is a tart and tasty option for cheese lovers—it's also lower in fat, calories, and cholesterol than many cow cheeses, such as cheddar.

1 CUP BOILING WATER

⅓ CUP SUNDRIED TOMATOES, PACKED WITHOUT OIL

2 TEASPOONS OLIVE OIL

½ CUP CHOPPED SHALLOTS, DIVIDED

1½ TEASPOONS SUGAR

3 GARLIC CLOVES, MINCED

2½ TABLESPOONS BALSAMIC VINEGAR, DIVIDED

½ CUP (ABOUT 2 OUNCES) CRUMBLED GOAT CHEESE

2 TABLESPOONS CHOPPED FRESH BASIL

¾ TEASPOON SALT

FOUR 6-OUNCE CHICKEN BREAST HALVES

⅛ TEASPOON FRESHLY GROUND PEPPER

¾ CUP FAT-FREE, LOW-SODIUM CHICKEN BROTH

¼ TEASPOON DRIED THYME

2 TEASPOONS CORNSTARCH

2 TEASPOONS WATER

1. In a small bowl, combine boiling water and tomatoes. Cover and let sit for 30 minutes, until soft. Drain and finely chop.

2. In a large nonstick skillet over medium heat, heat 1 teaspoon oil. Sauté ⅓ cup shallots, sugar, and garlic for 4 minutes, until golden brown. In a large mixing bowl, combine shallot mixture with 1½ teaspoons vinegar. Stir in chopped tomatoes, cheese, basil, and ¼ teaspoon salt, until well combined.

3. Using a paring knife or steak knife, cut a horizontal slit into the thickest part of each chicken breast half. Stuff each slit with about 2 tablespoons of tomato mixture. Season chicken with salt and pepper.

4. In a large nonstick skillet over medium-high heat, heat remaining 1 teaspoon oil. Cook chicken for 6 minutes on each side, or until cooked through. Remove chicken from heat. In the same pan, add broth, thyme, and remaining shallots and vinegar; bring to a boil. In a small bowl, whisk together cornstarch and water. Add cornstarch mixture to pan; bring to a boil. Cook 1 minute, whisking constantly, until sauce slightly thickens. Pour sauce over chicken and serve.

Mediterranean Chicken-Stuffed Pita Pockets

SERVES 4

▶ 330 CALORIES PER SERVING

▶ TOTAL PREPARATION TIME: 25 MINUTES

Even if you don't get the grill going for this dish, you'll still enjoy great flavors if you opt to cook the chicken in your kitchen. The lemony cucumber topping gives the sandwich a bright, fresh bite, while the savory yogurt dressing provides an indulgent creamy finish.

1 CUP PLAIN NONFAT GREEK YOGURT

2 TABLESPOONS PACKED FRESH MINT, CHOPPED

2 TABLESPOONS CHOPPED FRESH DILL

¾ TEASPOON GROUND CUMIN, DIVIDED

1 GARLIC CLOVE, CRUSHED, DIVIDED

½ TEASPOON PLUS A PINCH OF SALT, DIVIDED

2 TABLESPOONS FRESH LEMON JUICE

4 TEASPOONS OLIVE OIL

¼ TEASPOON DRIED OREGANO

1 POUND CHICKEN BREAST TENDERS

½ ENGLISH CUCUMBER, DICED

1 LARGE TOMATO, DICED

4 WHOLE-WHEAT PITAS, SPLIT IN HALF

1. Preheat either an outdoor grill or a grill pan to medium heat.

2. In a small mixing bowl, mix together yogurt, mint, dill, ¼ teaspoon cumin, one-third of the garlic, and ¼ teaspoon salt. Set aside.

3. In a large mixing bowl, combine 1 tablespoon lemon juice, 3 teaspoons oil, oregano, ¼ teaspoon salt, remaining ½ teaspoon cumin, and half of the remaining garlic. Add chicken to bowl and combine until well coated.

4. Grill chicken for about 5 minutes on each side, until cooked through.

5. As the chicken grills, use a large bowl to mix together cucumber, tomato, pinch of salt, remaining 1 tablespoon lemon juice, remaining 1 teaspoon oil, and remaining garlic.

6. When chicken is no longer pink, transfer to platter. Grill pitas until lightly toasted on both sides.

7. To assemble sandwiches, divide chicken among 4 pitas. Spoon in cucumber mixture and top with yogurt sauce.

Prosciutto-Wrapped Chicken

SERVES 4

▶ 202 CALORIES PER SERVING
▶ TOTAL PREPARATION TIME: 19 MINUTES

While fresh herbs can often be substituted with dried ones, it would be a shame to miss out on the taste of sage in this dish. The earthy herb truly shines as one of the main components. Also, try to stick to low-sodium chicken broth, as suggested— the prosciutto already adds plenty of salt to the meal.

FOUR 4-OUNCE CHICKEN CUTLETS
⅛ TEASPOON SALT
12 FRESH SAGE LEAVES
2 OUNCES THINLY SLICED PROSCIUTTO, DIVIDED INTO 8 THIN STRIPS
2 TABLESPOONS OLIVE OIL, DIVIDED
⅓ CUP FAT-FREE, LOW-SODIUM CHICKEN BROTH
¼ CUP FRESH LEMON JUICE
½ TEASPOON CORNSTARCH
LEMON WEDGES (OPTIONAL)

1. Season the chicken with salt. Line up three sage leaves on one side of each cutlet; secure the sage by wrapping each cutlet with 2 slices of prosciutto.

2. In a large skillet, heat 1 tablespoon oil over medium heat. Place chicken in pan and cook each side for 2 minutes. Remove chicken from skillet; keep warm.

3. In a small mixing bowl, whisk together the broth, lemon juice, and cornstarch until smooth. In the same skillet that you used for the chicken, add broth mixture and remaining oil. Bring to a boil, whisking constantly. Continue to cook for 1 minute, whisking constantly, until sauce is slightly thick. Spoon sauce over prepared chicken. Serve with lemon wedges (if using).

Sausage and Chicken Jambalaya

SERVES 4

▶ 341 CALORIES PER SERVING
▶ TOTAL PREPARATION TIME: 45 MINUTES

This Creole-inspired recipe will be full of flavor from the get-go, but consider making it the day before you're ready to eat it. After the flavors have time to meld, the dish will truly sing.

2 TEASPOONS CANOLA OIL
6 OUNCES REDUCED-FAT SMOKED CHICKEN SAUSAGE, HALVED
    LENGTHWISE AND CUT INTO ¼-INCH SLICES
½ CUP CHOPPED ONION
½ CUP CHOPPED CELERY
½ CUP CHOPPED GREEN BELL PEPPER
2 GARLIC CLOVES, MINCED
1 CUP UNCOOKED LONG-GRAIN WHITE RICE
1 CUP WATER
¼ TEASPOON GROUND RED PEPPER
⅛ TEASPOON SALT
6 FRESH THYME SPRIGS
ONE 14.5-OUNCE CAN FAT-FREE, LOW-SODIUM CHICKEN BROTH
ONE 14.5-OUNCE CAN NO-SALT-ADDED DICED TOMATOES, UNDRAINED
1 CUP SHREDDED ROTISSERIE CHICKEN BREAST

In a Dutch oven or heavy saucepan, heat oil over medium heat. Sauté sausage for 1 minute, until browned. Stir in onion, celery, bell pepper, and garlic; cook for 6 minutes, until softened. Mix in rice, water, red pepper, salt, thyme, and chicken broth; bring to a boil. Reduce heat, cover, and simmer for 20 minutes, until rice is cooked. Stir in tomatoes and chicken; cook for 3 minutes, until heated through. Discard thyme sprigs before serving.

Open-Faced Turkey and Havarti Sandwich with Sliced Apples

SERVES 4

▶ 427 CALORIES PER SERVING
▶ TOTAL PREPARATION TIME: 10 MINUTES

The combination of sweet apples, tangy Havarti, and peppery arugula makes this sandwich a real palate pleaser. If you're not one for mustard, feel free to omit it from this recipe—the sandwich is delicious with or without it.

4 SLICES BREAD
4 TEASPOONS LOW-FAT MAYONNAISE
4 TEASPOONS DIJON MUSTARD
1 CUP ARUGULA
FOUR ⅛-INCH-THICK SLICES RED ONION
12 OUNCES THINLY SLICED DELI TURKEY
2 APPLES, EACH CORED AND CUT CROSSWISE
    INTO EIGHT ¼-INCH-THICK SLICES
½ CUP (2 OUNCES) GRATED HAVARTI CHEESE
FRESHLY GROUND PEPPER

1. Preheat broiler.

2. Arrange sandwiches by spreading 1 teaspoon mayonnaise and 1 teaspoon mustard on each slice of bread. Add layers of ¼ cup arugula, 1 onion slice, 3 ounces turkey, 4 apple slices, and 2 tablespoons cheese on each.

3. Using a spatula, transfer sandwiches to a baking sheet. Broil for 4 minutes, until cheese is bubbly. Remove from heat and finish with a dash of pepper. Serve immediately.

Turkey Burgers with Sautéed Teriyaki Onions

SERVES 4

▶ 278 CALORIES PER SERVING
▶ TOTAL PREPARATION TIME: 35 MINUTES

Lighten up a classic burger by swapping out ground beef for ground turkey. For traditionalists who think turkey doesn't have enough flavor, this recipe works in sweet and savory onions that are a tasty addition to the meal.

1 POUND GROUND TURKEY BREAST

2 TEASPOONS GARLIC POWDER

1 TEASPOON CAJUN SEASONING

¼ TEASPOON FRESHLY GROUND PEPPER

3 TABLESPOONS LIGHT TERIYAKI SAUCE

1 TABLESPOON WATER

COOKING SPRAY

1 LARGE ONION, CUT INTO ¼-INCH SLICES

1 TEASPOON OLIVE OIL

4 HAMBURGER BUNS

EIGHT ¼-INCH SLICES OF TOMATO

4 LETTUCE LEAVES

1. In a large mixing bowl, combine ground turkey, garlic powder, Cajun seasoning, and pepper. Form 4 patties out of the mixture.

2. In a small bowl, whisk together teriyaki sauce and water.

3. Coat a large nonstick skillet with cooking spray, and heat pan over medium heat. Cover the skillet and sauté onions for 10 minutes. Mix in 1 tablespoon diluted teriyaki sauce. Remove onions from pan; set aside.

continued ▶

4. Using the same skillet, heat oil over medium heat. Cook the turkey patties for 5 minutes on each side. Spoon remaining 3 tablespoons diluted teriyaki sauce into the pan. Using a spatula, flip patties over; cook for 3 minutes, until lightly browned.

5. To assemble burgers, place 1 patty on each bottom bun. Top each with ¼ cup sautéed onion, 2 tomato slices, and 1 lettuce leaf. Finish with top of bun.

Rosemary-Garlic Pork Tenderloin

SERVES 4

▶ 147 CALORIES PER SERVING
▶ TOTAL PREPARATION TIME: 30 MINUTES

If you're growing tired of chicken breasts, there are plenty of other lean protein options out there. Pork tenderloin is a relatively budget-friendly alternative and "the other white meat" tends to be tender and juicy, if cooked with care. As this recipe proves, you only need a handful of ingredients to pack the pork with great flavor.

2 TABLESPOONS FINELY CHOPPED FRESH ROSEMARY
4 GARLIC CLOVES, MINCED
1 POUND PORK TENDERLOIN, TRIMMED
½ TEASPOON SALT
¼ TEASPOON FRESHLY GROUND PEPPER
COOKING SPRAY

1. Preheat oven to 475°F.

2. In a small bowl, combine the rosemary and garlic. Using a paring knife or steak knife, cut several slits into the pork loin. Stuff the slits with half of the garlic mixture. Rub the remaining garlic mixture around the pork loin. Season with salt and pepper. Coat a jelly roll pan or baking sheet with non-stick cooking spray. Place the tenderloin on the pan and insert an oven-safe meat thermometer into its thickest part.

3. Bake for 20 minutes or until tenderloin is slightly pink. The meat thermometer should read about 160°F. Remove tenderloin from oven and let it rest for 5 minutes before slicing.

Pork Chops with Mustard-Caper Sauce

SERVES 4

▶ 491 CALORIES PER SERVING
▶ TOTAL PREPARATION TIME: 30 MINUTES

This recipe proves that a delicious sauce can be made quickly, without butter or flour, and with only a few ingredients. The briny capers, tangy mustard, and aromatic rosemary come together for a savory and satisfying complement to the pork. Feel free to drizzle some extra sauce over steamed vegetables to enliven a simple side.

1 TABLESPOON OLIVE OIL
4 BONE-IN PORK LOIN CHOPS (ABOUT 3½ POUNDS TOTAL),
   ABOUT 1 INCH THICK
½ TEASPOON SALT
½ TEASPOON FRESHLY GROUND PEPPER
2 CUPS LOW-SODIUM CHICKEN BROTH
1½ TABLESPOONS WHOLE-GRAIN MUSTARD
3 TABLESPOONS CAPERS, RINSED
¼ TEASPOON CHOPPED FRESH ROSEMARY

1. In a large frying pan, heat oil over medium heat. Season pork with salt and pepper on both sides. Cook chops for 10 minutes on each side, until barely pink in the center. Transfer chops to serving dish.

2. In the same pan, pour in broth and bring to a boil over high heat. Mix in mustard, capers, and rosemary. Turn heat down; simmer sauce until it reduces by half, about 4 minutes. Pour sauce over pork and serve.

Meatballs with Tricolored Peppers

SERVES 4

▶ 263 CALORIES PER SERVING
▶ TOTAL PREPARATION TIME: 30 MINUTES

This recipe calls for ground round steak, which is about 85 percent lean. It's not as lean as sirloin—which is about 90 percent lean—but the negligible difference in fat will make for juicier meatballs. Also, you may replace the slice of whole-wheat bread with store-bought bread crumbs to save yourself some time.

1 CUP THINLY SLICED GREEN BELL PEPPER

1 CUP THINLY SLICED RED BELL PEPPER

1 CUP THINLY SLICED YELLOW BELL PEPPER

1⅓ CUPS PLUS ¼ CUP WATER

ONE 10.5-OUNCE CAN BEEF BROTH

1 BAY LEAF

1 SLICE WHOLE-WHEAT BREAD

1 POUND GROUND ROUND STEAK

1 TABLESPOON FINELY CHOPPED ONION

½ TEASPOON DRIED OREGANO

½ TEASPOON SALT

½ TEASPOON FRESHLY GROUND PEPPER

1 EGG WHITE

1 GARLIC CLOVE, CRUSHED

2 TEASPOONS OLIVE OIL

2 TABLESPOONS ALL-PURPOSE FLOUR

⅓ CUP FINELY CHOPPED FRESH BASIL (OR 1½ TEASPOONS DRIED)

2 TEASPOONS WHITE WINE VINEGAR

continued ▶

1. In a large saucepan, combine the bell peppers, 1⅓ cups water, broth, and bay leaf. Bring to a boil; cover and reduce heat. Simmer for 20 minutes.

2. While the peppers cook, use a food processor to pulse the bread, creating about ½ cup of coarse crumbs. In a large bowl, combine bread crumbs, beef, onion, oregano, salt, pepper, egg white, and garlic until well mixed. Shape beef mixture into 1-inch meatballs; the recipe should yield about 36.

3. In a large nonstick skillet, heat oil over medium-high heat. Cook meatballs for about 10 minutes, until they have browned on all sides.

4. In a small bowl, whisk together flour and remaining water. Pour flour mixture over peppers in saucepan and stir together. Add meatballs to pan; cook for 3 minutes, stirring constantly. Remove bay leaf; mix in basil and vinegar. Serve immediately.

Beef Sliders with Pita and Hummus

SERVES 4

▶ 488 CALORIES PER SERVING
▶ TOTAL PREPARATION TIME: 15 MINUTES

For a twist on the sliders craze, this dish pairs mini ground beef patties with a healthy serving of hummus. Make this dish even more Mediterranean by serving alongside a simple bed of romaine dressed with red wine vinegar and a light drizzle of olive oil, with a few feta crumbles on top.

1 POUND LEAN GROUND BEEF
1½ TEASPOONS DRIED OREGANO
SALT AND FRESHLY GROUND PEPPER
2 TABLESPOONS OLIVE OIL
4 POCKETLESS PITAS
¾ CUP STORE-BOUGHT HUMMUS
¼ SMALL RED ONION, CUT INTO THIN SLICES
2 TABLESPOONS FLAT-LEAF PARSLEY
LEMON WEDGES

1. Divide the beef into 16 half-inch-thick mini patties. Season with oregano, salt, and pepper.

2. In a large nonstick skillet, heat 1 tablespoon oil over medium heat. Cook patties for 2 minutes on each side, or until desired doneness.

3. To assemble the pitas, divide hummus among them and spread evenly. Layer 4 patties across each pita; top with onions and parsley. Finish each pita with a drizzle of oil and serve with a lemon wedge.

Stir-Fried Beef with Avocado and Black Bean Salad

SERVES 4

▶ 436 CALORIES PER SERVING
▶ TOTAL PREPARATION TIME: 10 MINUTES

Stir-frying your meat and vegetables is a quick way of preparing a one-pot, healthful dinner. This recipe calls for Cotija cheese, which is a dry, salty, sharp Mexican cheese that can be substituted with Parmesan or Asiago.

12 OUNCES BEEF TENDERLOIN, SLICED INTO THIN STRIPS
¼ CUP FRESH LIME JUICE, DIVIDED
1 TABLESPOON PLUS ½ TEASPOON CHILI POWDER
1 TABLESPOON VEGETABLE OIL
1 MEDIUM SWEET ONION, THINLY SLICED
1 RED BELL PEPPER, SEEDED, DERIBBED, AND THINLY SLICED
1 POBLANO PEPPER, SEEDED, DERIBBED, AND THINLY SLICED
½ TEASPOON SALT
½ TEASPOON FRESHLY GROUND PEPPER
ONE 15-OUNCE CAN BLACK BEANS, RINSED AND DRAINED
1 AVOCADO, DICED
¼ CUP CRUMBLED COTIJA CHEESE
¼ CUP CHOPPED FRESH CILANTRO

1. In a large mixing bowl, combine beef, 2 tablespoons lime juice, and 1 tablespoon chili powder; set aside.

2. In a large nonstick skillet, heat oil over medium heat. Sauté onion, bell pepper, and poblano for 5 minutes, stirring occasionally. Mix in beef and cook for 3 minutes. Season with salt and pepper.

3. In another mixing bowl, stir together beans, avocado, cheese, cilantro, remaining lime juice, and remaining ½ teaspoon chili powder. Serve salad alongside beef and vegetables.

Sliced Flank Steak with Balsamic Tomato Sauce

SERVES 4

▶ 246 CALORIES PER SERVING
▶ TOTAL PREPARATION TIME: 20 MINUTES

While certain cuts of meat can wreak havoc on a calorie-restricted menu, flank steak is a lean and relatively low-calorie pick for a healthy regimen. This dish will prove to be delicious year-round, but will be a standout during the summer months, when basil and tomatoes are at their prime.

1 TABLESPOON OLIVE OIL
1 POUND FLANK STEAK, TRIMMED
½ TEASPOON SALT
½ TEASPOON FRESHLY GROUND PEPPER
3 GARLIC CLOVES, MINCED
1 SHALLOT, MINCED
¼ CUP BALSAMIC VINEGAR
2 CUPS CHERRY TOMATOES, QUARTERED
⅓ CUP CHOPPED FRESH BASIL, DIVIDED
⅓ CUP THINLY SLICED GREEN ONIONS, DIVIDED

1. In a large skillet, heat oil over medium heat. Season steak with salt and pepper. Cook steak in pan for 5 minutes on each side, or until cooked to desired doneness. Remove steak from heat; transfer to a cutting board. Let it rest for 5 minutes before slicing thinly against the grain.

2. Meanwhile, use the same pan to sauté garlic and shallot over medium heat. Cook for 1 to 2 minutes, until lightly browned. Pour in vinegar and cook for 1 to 2 minutes, until liquid is almost fully reduced. Stir in tomatoes, ¼ cup basil, and ¼ cup green onions. Cook for 2 minutes, stirring occasionally. Once tomatoes have softened, pour mixture over steak. Finish with remaining basil and onions, and serve immediately.

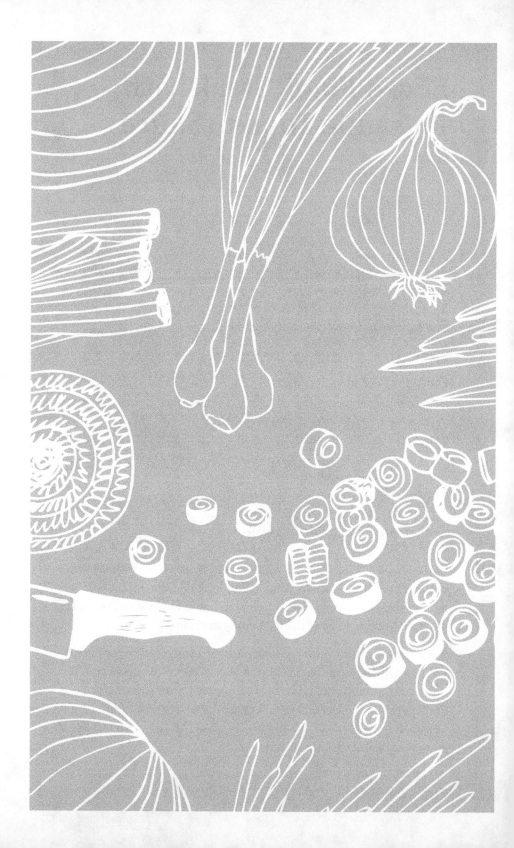

Dining Out

The 5:2 Diet is very flexible. You can schedule your fast days around any time you need to dine out. But sometimes plans change, and you may find yourself eating at a restaurant on a fast day. So it's good to have a few strategies for selecting menu items. Consider choosing:

- Simple salads with the dressing on the side and without croutons, cheese, or avocado
- Steamed, poached, baked, or grilled dishes—avoid menu selections described as pan-fried, battered, breaded, au gratin, deep fried, creamy, or crispy
- Menu items without sauces, toppings, or marinades
- Chicken breast (skinless), pork tenderloin, or fish
- Egg-white dishes
- Wraps with lean meats and vegetables
- Meals off the kids menu
- Meals seasoned with salsa, mustard, or flavored vinegars
- Side dishes, or ask for half of your meal to be wrapped up before it is served
- Foods prepared with olive oil instead of butter or shortening

No matter what meal you are eating in a restaurant you can substitute lower-calorie choices for some of your favorite dishes. Most restaurants are quite aware of dietary limitations, so make sure you tell your server that you need low-calorie and low-fat recommendations. Most restaurants are willing to accommodate your requests. Keep in mind that individual restaurants use different recipes for the items on their menu, so the following substitution chart is useful as a guide. A good tip: Try and order first so that your choices aren't affected by what everyone else orders. Studies have shown that people often duplicate orders in restaurant situations because of a desire to conform socially. Some good alternatives for higher-calorie restaurant fare include:

Regular Menu Item	Lower-Calorie Alternative
1 glass (6 ounces) white wine (135 calories)	1 gin and tonic (low calorie) (50 calories)
1 can coke (135 calories)	1 can diet coke (0 calories)
Café latte (200 calories)	Nonfat cappuccino (80 calories)
Whole-wheat banana muffin (430 calories)	Multigrain waffles (160 calories)
Blueberry muffin (550 calories)	½ bagel with low-sugar blueberry jam (165 calories)
Guacamole with tortilla chips (315 calories)	Salsa with baked tortilla chips (150 calories)
4-inch piece French bread (220 calories)	Whole-wheat roll (115 calories)
1 slice cheese pizza (450 calories)	1 slice cheese-less vegetable pizza (250 calories)
Cheese/onion quiche (595 calories)	Cheese/onion omelet (345 calories)
Baked potato with cheese (445 calories)	Baked potato with cottage cheese (335 calories)
Beef lasagna (665 calories)	Vegetarian lasagna (425 calories)
Pasta with a creamy carbonara sauce (1,020 calories)	Pasta with a tomato sauce (400 calories)
Cream of mushroom soup (270 calories)	Minestrone (126 calories)
Large chili (12 ounces), with cheese and sour cream (547 calories)	Small chili, 8 ounces (210 calories)
Fried chicken sandwich (570 calories)	Grilled chicken sandwich (380 calories)

Regular Menu Item	Lower-Calorie Alternative
French fries, medium (360 calories)	Baked potato (121 calories)
Chicken "nuggets" or tenders, 4 (240 calories)	Grilled chicken tenders, 4, (125 calories)
Caesar salad (390 calories)	Garden salad, without dressing (34 calories)
General Tso's chicken, 1 cup (296 calories)	Shrimp chow mein, 1 cup (143 calories)
Fried rice, 1 cup (333 calories)	Steamed brown rice, 1 cup (210 calories)

Low-Calorie Substitutes

Regular Food	Lower-Calorie Substitutes
Bacon or sausage	Canadian peameal back bacon or lean ham
Beef (chuck, rib, brisket)	Beef, trimmed of fat (round, loin)
Beef (regular ground)	Beef (extra lean); extra-lean ground turkey, chicken, or pork
Cheese	Reduced-calorie and low-fat cheese
Chicken or turkey with skin	Chicken or turkey (breast) without skin
Coffee creamer	Evaporated milk
Cream cheese	Light cream cheese or Neufchatel
Cream of chicken soup	Chicken noodle soup
Croissants	Multigrain dinner rolls
Eggs (whole)	Egg whites or egg substitute
Guacamole	Salsa
Hoisin sauce	Oyster sauce
Ice cream	Light ice cream, frozen yogurt, sorbet, granita
Mayonnaise (regular)	Mayonnaise (fat-free), mustard
Milk (regular)	Skim milk, 1% milk, or 2% milk

Regular Food	Lower-Calorie Substitutes
New England clam chowder	Manhattan clam chowder
Olive oil	Olive oil spray
Pork (spareribs, roast, chops)	Pork tenderloin, trimmed or lean smoked ham
Pasta with cheese sauce or white sauce	Pasta primavera or pasta with tomato sauce
Puddings (whole milk)	Puddings (skim milk) or fat-free
Salad dressings (regular)	Salad dressings (fat-free) or lemon juice
Sour cream	Sour cream (fat-free), yogurt, fat-free yogurt
Tuna (oil packed)	Tuna (water packed)

Calories of Popular Foods

Food	Portion	Calories
Alfalfa sprouts	1 cup	10
Almonds, whole	1 ounce	165
Applesauce, unsweetened	1 cup	105
Apples, unpeeled, 2 per pound	1	125
Apples, unpeeled, 3 per pound	1	80
Apricots, dried, unsweetened, cooked	1 cup	210
Apricots, dried, uncooked	1 cup	310
Apricots, raw	3	50
Asparagus, cooked from raw	1 cup	45
Asparagus, cooked from raw	4 spears	15
Avocados, Florida	1	340
Bagel, plain	1	200
Bananas	1	105
Barley, pearled, light and uncooked	1 cup	700
Bean sprouts	1 cup	25
Beef, ground 95% lean	3 ounces	115
Beef roast, lean	2.6 ounces	135
Beets	1 cup	59

Food	Portion	Calories
Beet greens, cooked	1 cup	40
Blackberries, raw	1 cup	75
Blueberries, raw	1 cup	80
Broccoli, raw	1 head	40
Brussels sprouts, raw	1 cup	60
Buttermilk	1 cup	100
Butter, salted	1 tablespoon	100
Cabbage, green, raw	1 cup	15
Cabbage, red, raw	1 cup	20
Cabbage, Savoy, raw	1 cup	20
Cantaloupe, raw	½ melon	95
Carrots, raw, baby	10 medium	30
Carrots, raw	1 whole	30
Cauliflower, raw	1 cup	25
Celery, raw	1 stalk	5
Cheddar cheese	1 ounce	115
Cherries, sweet, raw	10	50
Chicken breast, roasted	3 ounces	140
Chickpeas, cooked	1 cup	270
Coffee, brewed	6 fluid ounces	0
Coffee, instant	6 fluid ounces	0
Collards, raw	1 cup	25
Corn, cooked from frozen	1 cup	135

Food	Portion	Calories
Corn, cooked from raw	1 ear	85
Cottage cheese, 2%	1 cup	205
Cracked-wheat bread	1 slice	65
Cranberries, dried	1 tablespoon	26
Cream cheese	1 ounce	100
Cream cheese, fat-free	1 ounce	28
Cream of wheat, cooked	1 package	100
Cucumber with peel	6 slices	5
Dates	10	230
Eggplant, cooked	1 cup	25
Eggs, whites, raw	1	15
Eggs, whole, raw	1	75
Eggs, yolk, raw	1	60
Endive, curly, raw	1 cup	10
English muffin, plain	1	140
Evaporated milk, canned	1 cup	200
Feta cheese, low calorie	¼ cup	60
Figs	1 medium	37
Filberts, chopped	1 ounce	180
Grapefruit, pink, raw	½ fruit	40
Grapefruit, white, raw	½ fruit	40
Grapes, red, raw	10	35
Grapes, green, raw	10	40

Food	Portion	Calories
Half–and–half cream	1 tablespoon	20
Honey	1 tablespoon	65
Honeydew melon, raw	1/10 melon	45
Jam	1 tablespoon	55
Kale, cooked from raw	1 cup	40
Kiwi	1	45
Lamb rib, roasted, lean	2 ounces	130
Lamb chops, roasted, lean	1.7 ounces	135
Lemons	1	15
Lemon juice	1 fruit's yield	20
Lentils, dried, cooked	1 cup	215
Lettuce, Boston, raw	1 head	20
Lettuce, looseleaf, raw	1 cup	10
Light table or coffee cream	1 tablespoon	30
Lima beans, dried, cooked	1 cup	260
Lime	1	20
Lime juice	1 cup	65
Mayonnaise, fat-free	1 tablespoon	40
Milk, low fat, 1%	1 cup	105
Milk, skim	1 cup	90
Mixed-grain bread	1 slice	65
Mozzarella cheese, full milk	1 ounce	80
Mushrooms, raw	1 cup	20

Food	Portion	Calories
Mustard greens, cooked from raw	1 cup	20
Mustard, yellow	1 tablespoon	5
Nectarines	1	65
Oatmeal, rolled, dry	⅓ cup	105
Oatmeal bread	1 slice	65
Olive oil	1 tablespoon	125
Onions, raw, chopped	1 cup	55
Oranges	1	60
Papaya, raw	1 cup	65
Parmesan cheese, grated	1 ounce	130
Parsnips, diced, raw	1 cup	125
Peaches	1	35
Peanut butter	1 tablespoon	95
Pears, Anjou, raw	1	120
Pears, Bosc, raw	1	85
Peas, edible pods	1 cup	65
Peppers, hot chili, raw	1	20
Peppers, green bell, raw	1	20
Peppers, red bell, raw	1	20
Pineapple, diced, raw	1 cup	75
Pistachios	1 ounce	165
Plums, 2 inch	1	15
Plums, 3 inch	1	35
Pork chop, lean	2.5 ounces	165

Food	Portion	Calories
Pork, back bacon	2 slices	85
Pork, cured ham	3 ounces	140
Pork tenderloin, lean	3 ounces	159
Potatoes, peeled	1	120
Pumpernickel bread	1 slice	80
Radishes, raw	4 radishes	5
Raisins, dried	.5 ounce	42
Raspberries, raw	1 cup	60
Red kidney beans, canned	1 cup	230
Rice, brown, cooked	1 cup	230
Rye bread, light	1 slice	65
Salmon, baked	3 ounces	140
Sesame seeds	1 tablespoon	45
Snap beans, green, raw	1 cup	45
Snap beans, yellow, raw	1 cup	45
Sour cream	1 tablespoon	25
Spaghetti, cooked	1 cup	190
Spinach, raw	1 cup	10
Squash, summer, raw	1 cup	35
Squash, winter, baked	1 cup	80
Strawberries, raw	1 cup	45
Sunflower seeds	1 ounce	160
Sweet chocolate, 70% dark	1 ounce	150

Food	Portion	Calories
Sweet potatoes, peeled, baked	1	115
Sweet potatoes, peeled, boiled	1	160
Tangerines	1	35
Tea, brewed	8 fluid ounces	0
Tofu	1 piece	85
Tomatoes, canned	1 cup	50
Tomatoes, raw	1	25
Tomatoes, raw, cherry	5	20
Tortillas, corn	1	65
Tuna, water packed	3 ounces	135
Turkey ham, lean	2 slices	75
Turkey, breast meat, roasted	2 pieces	135
Turnips, diced, cooked	1 cup	30
Vinegar, cider	1 tablespoon	0
Watermelon, 1 piece, raw	1 piece	155
Watermelon, diced, raw	1 cup	50
Wheat bread	1 slice	65
Whole-wheat bread	1 slice	70
Yogurt with low-fat milk, plain	8 ounces	145
Yogurt with nonfat milk, plain	8 ounces	125

References

Allard, Joanne S., Evelyn Perez, Sige Zou, and Rafael de Cabo. 2009. "Dietary activators of Sirt1." *Molecular and Cellular Endocrinology*, 299 (1): 58–63.

Brown, James E., Michael Mosley, and Sarah Aldred. 2013. "Intermittent fasting: A dietary intervention for prevention of diabetes and cardiovascular disease." *British Journal of Diabetes and Vascular Disease*, 13 (2): 68–72.

Fontana, L., Timothy E. Meyer, Samuel Klein, and John O. Holloszy. 2004. "Long-term calorie restriction is highly effective in reducing the risk for atherosclerosis in humans." *Proceedings of the National Academy of Sciences*, 101 (17): 6659–6663.

Fontana, Luigi, Edward P. Weiss, Dennis T. Villareal, Samuel Klein, and John O. Holloszy. 2008. "Long-term effects of calorie or protein restriction on serum IGF-1 and IGFBP-3 concentration in humans." *Aging Cell*, 7 (5): 681–87.

Harvie, M., C. Wright, M. Pegington, D. McMullan, E. Mitchell, B. Martin, R. G. Cutler, G. Evans, S. Whiteside, S. Maudsley, S. Camandola, R. Wang, O. D. Carlson, J. M. Egan, M. P. Mattson, and A. Howell. 2013. "The effect of intermittent energy and carbohydrate restriction v. daily energy restriction on weight loss and metabolic disease risk markers in overweight women." *British Journal of Medicine*, 110 (8): 1534–47.

Hughes, T. A., J. T. Gwynne, B. R. Switzer, C. Herbst, and G. White. 1984. "Effects of caloric restriction and weight loss on glycemic control, insulin release and resistance, and atherosclerotic risk in obese patients with type II diabetes mellitus." *American Journal of Medicine*, 717.

Kraemer, Frederic B., and Wen-Jun Shen. 2002. "Hormone-sensitive lipase control of intracellular tri-(di-)acylglycerol and cholesteryl ester hydrolysis." *Journal of Lipid Research*, 43 (10): 1585–94.

Longo, Lee C. 2011. "Fasting vs. dietary restriction in cellular protection and cancer treatment: From model organisma to patients." *Oncogene*, 3305–16.

Mattson, M. P., and R. Wan. 2005. "Beneficial effects of intermittent fasting and caloric restriction on the cardiovascular and cerebrovascular systems." *Journal of Nutritional Biochemistry*, 16 (3): 129–37.

Nematy, Mohsen, Maryann Alinezhad-Namaghi, Masoud Mahdavi Rashed, Mostafa Mozhdehifard, Seyedeh Sania Sajjadi, Saeed Akhlaghi, Maryam Sabery, Seyed Amir R. Mohajeri, Neda Shalaey, Mohsen Moohebati, and Abdolreza Norouzy. 2012. "Effects of Ramadan fasting on cardiovascular risk factors: A prospective observational study." *Nutrition Journal*, September 2010 (11): 69.

Raffaghello, Lizzia, Fernando Safdie, Giovanna Bianchi, Tanya Dorff, Luigi Fontana, and Valter D. Longo. 2010. "Fasting and differential chemotherapy protection in patients." *Cell Cycle*, 9 (22): 4474–76.

Sohal, R. S., and R. Weindruch. 1996. "Oxidative stress, caloric restriction, and aging." *Science*, 273 (5271): 59–63.

Duan, Wenzhen, Zhilong Guo, Haiyang Jiang, Melvin Ware, Xiao-Jiang Li, and Mark P. Mattson. 2003. "Dietary restriction normalizes glucose metabolism and BDNF levels, slows disease progression, and increases survival in Huntington mutant mice." *Proceedings of the National Academy of Sciences*, 100 (5): 2911–16.

Index